The 21-Day Meal Plan Anti-Inflammatory Diet

The Comprehensive Guide And Easy To Follow Recipes To Boost The Immune System. A No-Stress Meal Plan To Reduce Inflammation And Rapid Weight Loss

By Dr. Al White

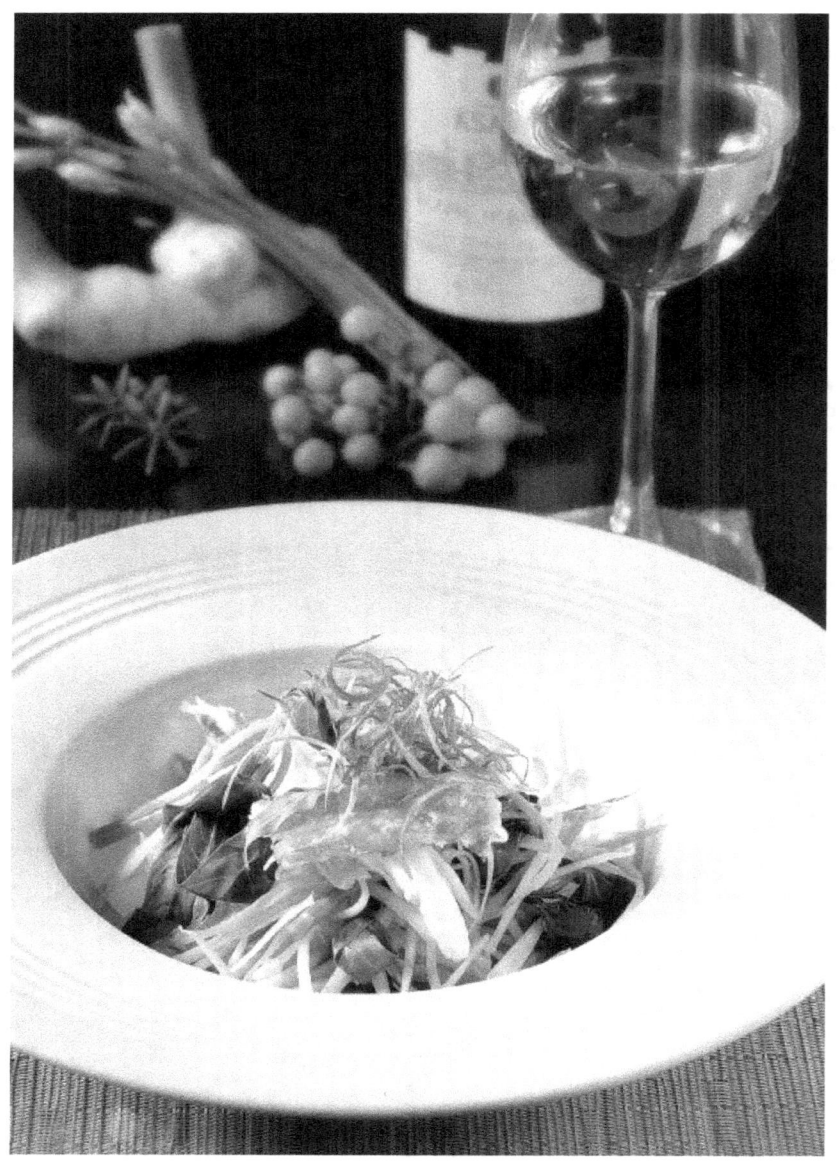

Contents

- INTRODUCTIONS 13
- WHAT IS ANTI INFLAMMATORY MEAL? 15
- ANTI INFLAMMATORY FOODS 16
- WHO SHOULD EAT INFLAMMATORY DIET? 19
- HOW ANTI INFLAMMATORY DIET WORKS 21
- WHAT IS INFLAMMATION ? 23
- SIDE EFFECTS OF INFLAMMATION 24
- WHY EXCESSIVE INFLAMMATION IS SO COMMON 26
- INFLAMMATION: WHO IS AT RISK? 27
- SCARCELY THINGS TO KNOW ABOUT INFLAMMATION ... 29
- ANTI-INFLAMMATORY DIET: SAMPLE MEAL PLAN 33
- ANTI-INFLAMMATORY DIETS: RULES FOR OPTIMAL HEALTH 34
- ADVANTAGES OF ANTI INFLAMMATORY DIETS 35
- TOP INFLAMMATION CURING FOOD 38
- CORE VALUE TO CHOOSING A MEAL PLAN 42
- BENEFITS OF REDUCING INFLAMMATION 43
- TOWARDS A BETTER INFLAMMATORY LIFESTYLE 43
- EXERCISE AND INFLAMMATION 48
- SELECTED EXERCISES TO REDUCE INFLAMMATION 49

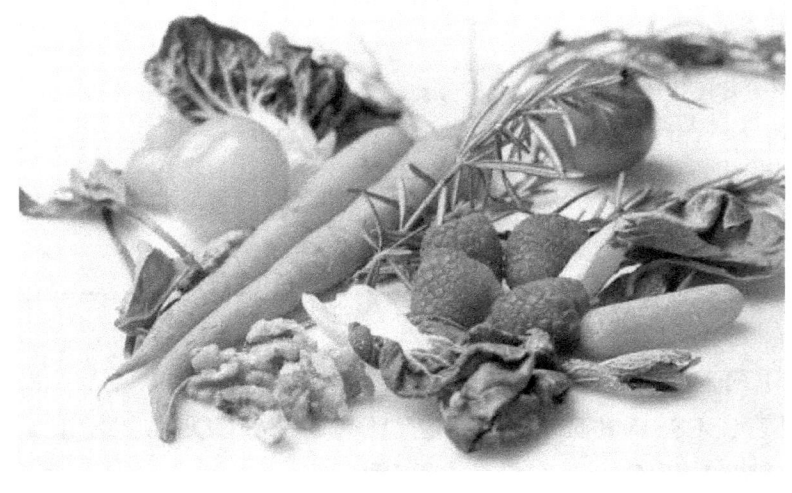

The 21-Day Meal Plan 52

Chapter 1 -Anti-Inflammatory: Breakfast Recipes 55
1. Oven-Poached Eggs 55
2. Breakfast Marinated Egg 56
3. Breakfast Omelette 57
4. Cranberry and Raisins Granola 57
5. Breakfast French Onion Soup 58
6. Spicy Marble Eggs 59
7. Nutty Oats Pudding 60
8. Couscous with Lettuce and Carrots Salad 61
9. Barley and Mushroom Soup 62
10. Almond Pancakes with Coconut Flakes 63

11. Cooled Almond Soup 64
12. Baked Apple Turnover 65
13. Quinoa and Cauliflower Congee 66
14. Breakfast ArrozCaldo 67
15. Fried Vegetable Brown Rice 68
16. Apple Bruschetta with Almonds and Blackberries 69
17. Hash Browns 69
18. Cucumber Jicama Salad with Cashew Butter 70
19. RomanescoSalad with Quail Eggs 71
20. Asparagus and Artichoke Salad with Dijon Vinaigrette 71
21. Barley Apple Salad 72
22. Cucumber and Pepper Salad 73
23. Potatoes and Leeks Soup 74
24. Sun-Dried Tomato Garlic Bruschetta 75
25. Mushroom Crêpes 75
Chapter 2 - Anti-Inflammatory: Lunch Recipes 77
26. Capellini Soup with Tofu and Shrimp 77
27. Chicken and Vegetable Salad with Hollandaise Sauce 78
28. Iceberg Lettuce and Mushrooms Salad 79
29. Arugula with Gorgonzola Dressing 79
30. Fusilli with Grape Tomatoes and Kale 80
31. Rice and Chicken Pot 81
32. Shiitake and SpinachPattie 82
33. Cabbage Orange Salad with Citrusy Vinaigrette 83
34. Lemon Buttery Shrimp Rice 83
35. Valencia Salad 84
36. Tenderloin Stir Fry with Red and Green Grapes 85
37. Aioli with Eggs 86

38. Aioli on Spaghetti Squash 86
39. Vegetable Noodle Salad with Raspberry Dressing.............. 87
40. Ginger Chicken Stew 88
41. Taro Leaves in Coconut Sauce 88
42. Buttered Prawns in Garlic Rice 89
43. Pesto Chicken Sandwich 90
44. Pepper Stuffed Quinoa 91
45. Mixed Veggies with Oregano Vinaigrette.......................... 92
46. All Seafood Stock 93
47. Seared Herbed Salmon Steak 93
48. Steamed Meatballs on Bed of Rice..................................... 94

Chapter 3 - Anti-Inflammatory: Dinner Recipes 96

49. Hot Dumpling Soup 96
50. Artichoke Hearts Crisps 98
51. Maple Turkey 98
52. Crab Avocado Cilantro Salad... 99
53. Chicken Barbeque Bake... 99
54. Mango Bell Pepper Salsa 100
55. Buttered Cauliflower Mash...101
56. Salmon and Pickle Salad 101
57. Garlic Lean Pork 102
58. OLIVES and Eggs Rollups.. 103
59. ASPARAGUS and Peppers Terrine 103
60. Mushrooms and Baby Onions... 104
61. Artichoke Soup.. 105
62. Courgettes and Peppers with Cashew Nuts 106
63. Salmon with Broccoli and Sweet Potato 107
64. Turkey Salad... 108

65. Zucchini Endive Soup 108
66. Unsalted Vegetable Broth 109
67. Spiced Mussel Broth 110
68. Hot Kiwi, Mango, Berries Salad 111
69. All Mushroom Soup 111
70. Tuna Salad Wrapped in Lettuce 112
71. Fish Egg Rolls 113
72. Veggie Rolls 114
73. Cabbage and Fish Egg Rolls 115
74. Pork Fillet Noodles 116
75. Chicken Noodle Soup 117
76. Zucchini, Kale, and Shrimp Noodles 118
77. Rice and Prawn Noodles 119
78. Rice Beef, and Prawns Noodles 119
79. Rice and Chicken Noodles 120
80. Egg and Mushrooms Bake 121
81. Spinach, Artichoke, and Pumpkin Seeds Casserole 122
82. Chicken Salad with Cabbage and Lettuce 123
83. Fish Stock with Ginger 123
84. Cucumber, Corn, and Bell Pepper Salad 124
85. Asian Chicken Salad 125
86. Mushroom Curry 126
87. Baked Stuffed Meatballs 127
88. Melon and Watermelon Salad 128
89. Beef Mushroom Soup 128
90. Chicken, Mushroom and Vegetable Soup 129
91. Creamy Chicken Curry 131
Chapter 4 - Anti-Inflammatory: Desserts & Snacks Recipes ... 132

92. Cherry Jam 132
93. Apricot Cinnamon Jam 133
94. Sautéed Apples 133
95. Protein Crepes 134
96. Banana Cinnamon Sandwich 135
97. Apple Parfait 135
98. Olive Crostini 136
99. Banana Cinnamon 137
100. Banana Cinnamon Cookies 138
101. Avocado Chia Parfait 138
102. Honeyed Sweet Potatoes 139
103. Banana Dark AlmondsChoco 140
104. Chocolate Avocado Pudding 141
105. Blueberry Pudding 141
106. Apple Chips 142
107. Baked Cinnamon Apples 143
108. Tapenade Crostini 144
109. Honey Baked Apricots 144
110. Crostiniwith Tomato Spread 145
111. Sweet Potatoes in Creamy Coconut Sauce 146
112. Honey Baked Apples with Walnuts 146
113. Dark Chocó Almond Butter 147
114. Sweet Potato and Chia Butter 148
115. Chia Bread 148
116. Crostini Arugula and Spinach 149
117. Pepper Pizza 150
118. Grilled Plantains 151
119. Sweet Potato Matchsticks 151

120. Cauliflower Poppers	152
121. Breaded Blossoms	153
122. Crostini Garlic	153
123. Chicken Enchiladas	154
124. Cashew Butter	156
125. Burritos	156
126. Tofu Patties	158
Chapter 5 - Anti-Inflammatory: Rare Slow Cooked Meals	159
127. Beef Borscht	159
128. Pork and Beef Spice	160
129. Creamy Pork Stew in Yogurt Sauce	161
130. Rum Pork Shoulder	162
131. Braised Pork Shanks	163
132. Stewing Beef with Horseradish Cream	164
133. King Prawn Curry	165
134. Cod Tagine	166
135. Lamb Bone Broth	167
136. Turkey Bone Broth	168
137. Odds and Ends Beef Stew	168
138. Swedish Meatballs	169
139. Savory Cocoa-Flavored Baby Back Ribs	170
140. Tuna in Brine	171
141. Seafood Stew	172
142. Veal Roast	173
143. Pork with Tomatoes	173
144. Balsamic Pork	174
145. Braised Brisket	175
146. Stewed Oxtails	176

147. Pot Roast 177
148. Oxtails with Celery 178
149. Italian- Style Goulash 178
150. Coco Ginger Linguine 180
151. Vegan Macaroni and Cheese 181
152. Glazed Salmon 182
153. Stroganoff 182
154. Barley and Squash Crockpot 183
155. Seitan in Tomato and Soy Yogurt 184
156. Cranberry-Apple Pork 185
157. Herbed Tenderloin 185
158. Corn and Mushroom 186
159. Thai Tofu Bowls 186
160. Beef with Mushrooms and Sweet Potato 187
CONCLUSION 189

© **Copyright 2020 - All rights reserved.**

The content contained within this book may not be reproduced, duplicated or transmitted without direct written permission from the author or the publisher.

Under no circumstances will any blame or legal responsibility be held against the publisher, or author, for any damages, reparation, or monetary loss due to the information contained within this book. Either directly or indirectly.

Legal Notice:

This book is copyright protected. This book is only for personal use. You cannot amend, distribute, sell, use, quote or paraphrase any part, or the content within this book, without the consent of the author or publisher.

Disclaimer Notice:

Please note the information contained within this document is for educational and entertainment purposes only. All effort has been executed to present accurate, up to date, and reliable, complete information. No warranties of any kind are declared or implied. Readers acknowledge that the author is not engaging in the rendering of legal, financial, medical or professional advice. The content within this book has been derived from various sources. Please consult a licensed professional before attempting any techniques outlined in this book.

By reading this document, the reader agrees that under no circumstances is the author responsible for any losses, direct or indirect, which are incurred as a result of the use of information contained within this document, including, but not limited to, — errors, omissions, or inaccuracies.

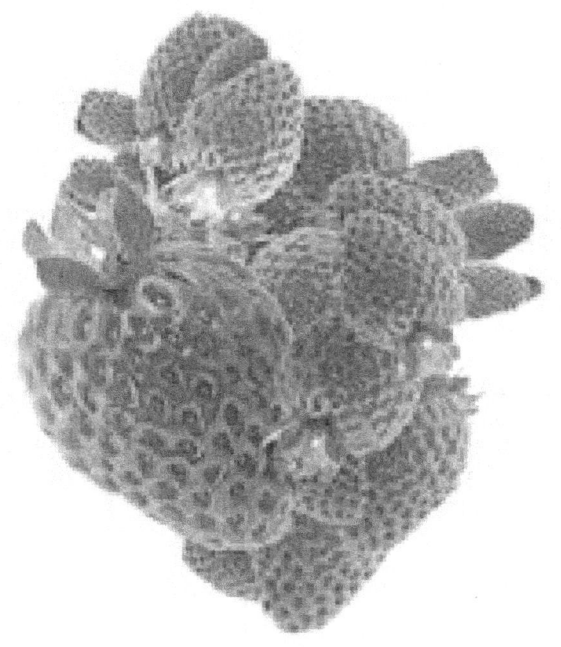

INTRODUCTIONS

The anti-inflammatory diet is grounded on a simple decree - chronic inflammation, which leads to a host of chronic illnesses. When you try to reduce inflammation through an anti-inflammatory diet, it can counteract diseases while promoting good health in such an unbelievable way.

An anti-inflammatory diet's goal is to encourage the ideal function of both the body and brain. If it does what it says, it is then possible to prevent the signs of Alzheimer's, heart disease, inflammatory bowel disease, different types of cancer, arthritis, diabetes, gout, and many more. However, the plan still consists of tasty foods. So much so, you won't believe you're on an actual diet. Better yet, you have positively taken your health to it's highest potential.

Acute inflammation is healthy and is essential for the body to experience. This may include times of injury, such as spraining your ankle or scraping your knee. The swelling and redness that comes with minor wounds is considered inflammation. However, chronic inflammation is different and harmful to the body. This can pave the way for many diseases to transpire. The anti-inflammatory diet, initially developed by Dr. Andrew Weil, is not a diet as it is popularly coined. Instead, it is a food recommendation done long term in order to attain and support prolonged optimum health. This experience has been the reason why the anti-inflammatory diet has been the most extensive practice amongst the modern western world.

Most people who experience inflammation have heard all about the medications that are available to cure the pain and swelling that can occur during a flare-up. However, how many know that some tremendous anti-inflammatory foods can affect how you feel and reduce the pain associated with inflammation. Following a JHU anti-inflammatory diet will help you beat inflammation naturally. That is why most medical practitioners who understand the essential benefits, also refer an inflammatory patient to this healthy mouth-watering diet.

Inflammation is a swelling that may cause pain, discoloration, and even the loss of movement. Usually, most people experience severe inflammation when they have arthritis, or more chronic issues like heart disease and strokes.

Usually, your doctor will recommend that you get some sleep and exercise in moderation. The doctor may also suggest losing weight, taking steroid-based drugs or undergoing joint replacement surgery. The medications do work reasonably well in reducing the inflammation, but often come with severe side effects, such as ulcers and kidney problems. This may make you fear whether they are worth having and whether using them is trading one illness for another serious issues.

Furthermore, just like there are some foods that decrease inflammation, some will increase the likelihood that you will get inflammation. These foods are junk foods, fast foods, sugars, and fatty meats. Processed foods that contain trans-fat and saturated fats also increase the risk of inflammation. Other large contributors of saturated fats are dairy products and eggs. By merely choosing low-fat milk, low-fat cheese, and leaner cuts of meat, you can lower the risk of inflammation, as well as cutting down the chances of developing chronic diseases and obesity. Some other foods that increase inflammation are pre-sweetened cereals, soft drinks and other processed items. In addition to these, some foods are high in sugar and foods that come from plants labelled as *nightshade* type. These add to the risk of discomfort associated with inflammation. Eating an anti-inflammatory diet like vegetables, will give you natural healing factors. However, not all herbs work that way. Potatoes, eggplant, and tomatoes can make inflammation worse.

Remember, the best foods to have are whole fruits, fresh vegetables, lean meats, low-fat milk and cheese; as well as fruit and vegetable juices that contain carrots and celery and many other vegetables. These types of foods will reduce inflammation and help you live your life without pain. Therefore, healthy eating will help you stop inflammation naturally.

Engage in any activity or sport that you enjoy the most. It could be tennis, golf, ballroom dancing, yoga, or any physical activity that pleases you. The bottom line is, you need to move around to get your legs, feet, muscles, and joints moving...and have some fun.

WHAT IS ANTI INFLAMMATORY MEAL?

An anti-inflammatory meal consists of foods that diminish inflammatory reactions. A diet that is anti-inflammatory contains expanded amounts of antioxidants, which are receptive molecules in food that lessen the number of free radicals. Free radicals harm cells and increase the danger of specific diseases.

    Numerous mainstream diets, as of now, pursue anti-inflammatory standards. Different foods are utilized in an unexpected way, some advancing inflammation and others decreasing it. The reason for the anti-inflammatory diet is to advance ideal wellbeing and mending, by picking foods that decrease inflammation. On the off chance that one can effectively control exorbitant inflammation through characteristic methods (like through diet); it diminishes one's reliance on anti-inflammatory medications that have undesirable and unfortunate symptoms, and do not tackle the hidden issue. While anti-inflammatory medications (for example, NSAIDs) are a handy solution to ease indications, they debilitate the safe framework by harming the gastrointestinal tract; which assumes a significant job in an invulnerable framework. When all is said and done, an anti-inflammatory diet consists of new, entire foods that do not contain triggers for inflammation, and are loaded with molecules that kill inflammation in your body.

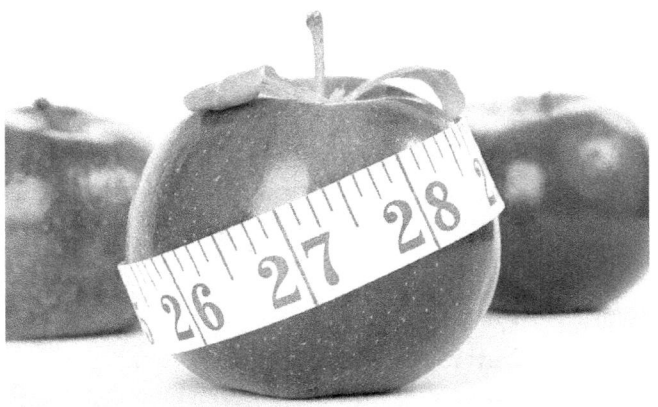

ANTI INFLAMMATORY FOODS

Inflammation has been distinguished as the reason for most chronic diseases like joint pain, stoutness, diabetes, coronary illness, and much malignant growth. It is hard to believe, but it is true. Most chronic diseases are an aftereffect of wealthy habits that bear us the advantage of having the option to eat inappropriate food, in an inappropriate amount, on inappropriate occasions. These food choices set in play a large group of procedures in your body that produce inflammation from a huge number of sources. Furthermore, an excessive number of us are hereditarily customized to produce extreme inflammation when presented to normal aggravation sources for example, smoke, synthetic concoctions, and poor dietary choices. A few of us produce so much inflammation, that we have immune system issues, such as: lupus, different sclerosis, rheumatoid joint inflammation, psoriasis, and colitis.

Foods that are rich in refined sugars are likewise inflammatory. Cakes, cookies, and doughnuts are types of food that are quickly processed by your body, discharging a lot of glucose. This glucose is instantly absorbed by your body, which causes a high blood glucose level. Your body thus releases a surge of insulin to help standardize your blood glucose levels. This surge of insulin joined with high blood glucose levels, makes your body release cytokines, inflammatory molecules, too. Each surge of glucose flags your body to store fat. *Prepare to have your mind blown.* Fat tissue turns out to be physiologically dynamic. It starts to release these equivalent inflammatory molecules, cytokines, too refined grains, grains deprived of fiber, and essential supplements that additionally make inflammation. An entire grain is a molecule made out of a lot of glucose connected and typified with a fiber coating. This fiber coating makes the absorption and release of glucose a gradual procedure. At the point when the external fiber coating is stripped away to make a smooth and rich surface, glucose molecules are promptly accessible for quick assimilation and ingestion into your body. This quick surge of glucose into your framework again is the trigger for the inflammatory course. Certain grains can produce inflammation in specific people. Wheat, oats, grain, and rye are, for the most part, grains that contain noteworthy amounts of a protein substance called gluten. Gluten makes foods, similar to bread, crunchy outwardly, and delicate within. However, this equivalent gluten is inflammatory in people hereditarily tested in processing gluten. Side effects can be as extreme as torment, swelling, looseness of the bowels and being unhealthy, or as mellow as queasiness, or absence of vitality. Disposing of these particular grains from your diet is frequently the way to controlling this sort of inflammation. Great choices for an individual after an anti-inflammatory diet integrate greens (kale and spinach), blueberries, blackberries, and fruits dull red grapes, nutrition-thick vegetables (broccoli and cauliflower, beans and lentils), green tea wine, with some restraint avocado and coconut olives additional virgin olive oil pecans, pistachios, pine nuts, and almonds. As well as cold-water fish, including salmon and sardines turmeric and cinnamon dim chocolate flavors and herbs. The fundamental foods that individuals following an anti-inflammatory diet ought to maintain a strategic distance from incorporate handled meats, sugary drinks, trans fats, found in singed foods, white bread, white pasta, gluten, soybean oil, and vegetable oil, prepared snack foods (chips and crackers) desserts (cookies, treat, and ice cream), excess liquor and such a large number of starches. There are a few things an individual can do to make progress to an anti-inflammatory diet simpler, including:

- Eating an assortment of products of the soil.
- Reducing the amount of inexpensive food eaten.
- Eliminating soft drink and sugary refreshments.
- Planning shopping records to guarantee invigorating dinners and snacks are close by.
- Carrying little anti-inflammatory snacks while in a hurry
- Drinking more water.
- Staying inside the everyday calorie necessities.
- Adding supplements, for example, omega-3 and turmeric, to the diet.
- Exercising routinely.
- Getting the best possible amount of rest.

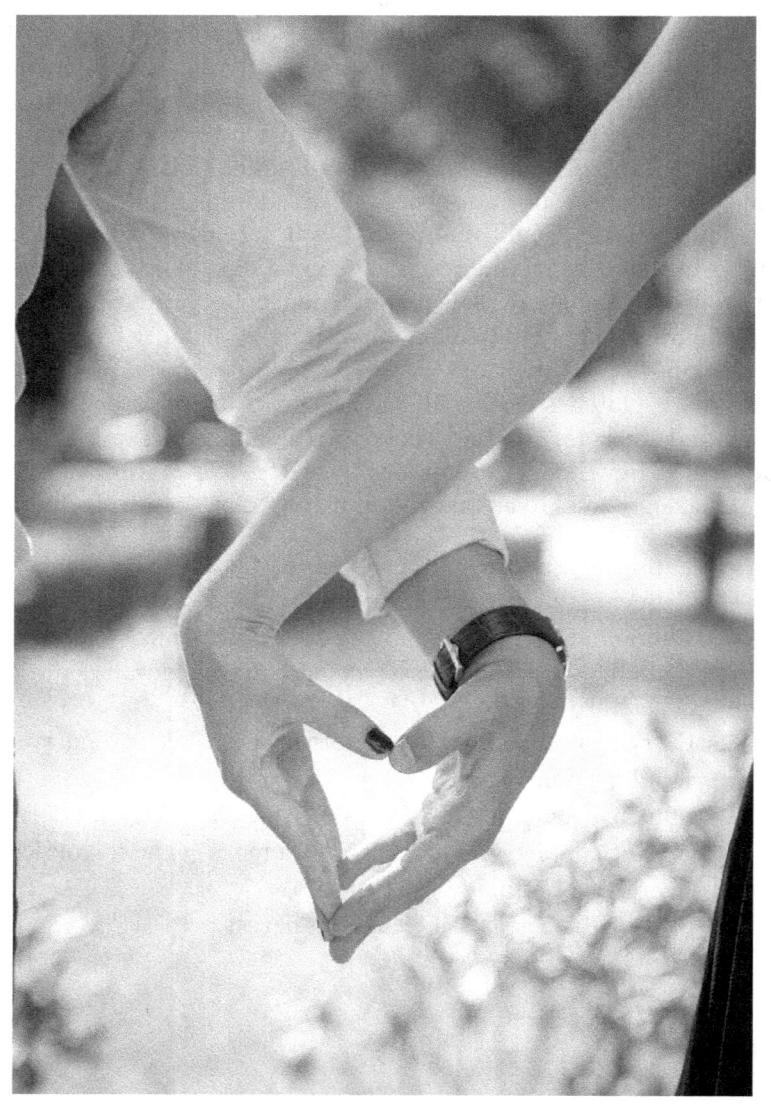

WHO SHOULD EAT INFLAMMATORY DIET?

Clearly, any individual who experiences an inflammatory condition, for example, immune system disorders (lupus, different sclerosis, rheumatoid arthritis, colitis, etc.) or hypersensitive disorders (asthma, skin inflammation), will benefit from the anti-inflammatory diet. A great many people with ceaseless pain (migraines, back, neck, knee, joint, nerve, muscle pains, etc.) have components of inflammation engaged with their pain and will benefit as well. Peevish entrails disorder and normal stomach related disorders, for example acid reflux, improve with the anti-inflammatory diet. However, shockingly, anybody enduring endless degenerative disorders (arthritis, diabetes, heart disease, corpulence, and many cancers) will also benefit from this diet. At last, anybody keen on anticipating these degenerative diseases and accomplishing ideal health will benefit. Indeed, the science affirms that eating to avoid inflammation forestalls disease and keeps up health, as well as keeps us looking and feeling more youthful. While a few foods appear to ease inflammation, mixes in others have been found to expand it. Eating burgers, chicken, or other meats that have been barbecued or broiled at a high temperature can raise the measure of innovative glycation finished results (AGEs) in the blood. Albeit, no immediate connection among AGEs and arthritis has been recognized, abnormal amounts of AGEs have been distinguished in people with inflammation.

Another guilty party that may support inflammation is omega-6 fatty acids, which are found in corn, sunflower, safflower and soybean oils, and many bites and browned foods. Expending more omega-6 fatty acids than omega-3s, raises your danger of joint inflammation and stoutness. Keep crisp fruits and veggies close by to enable you to stay away from handled tidbits that regularly contain omega-6 fatty acids. Because of menopause or steroid treatment, a few people with RA may require a greater amount of specific vitamins and minerals. The most widely recognized lacks are in folic acid, vitamins C, D, B6, B12 and E, calcium, magnesium, selenium, and zinc. Nutritionists concur that most supplements should originate from your food, rather than from enhancements. Once again, discuss with your doctor before taking any enhancement. The primary concern when considering sustenance and RA, is to keep up a healthy, well-adjusted diet. One way to accomplish this is to consider receiving a Mediterranean diet, which incorporates many omega-3 fatty acids, fruits, vegetables, and entire grains, the benefits of olive oil or even a glass of red wine, if your doctor permits.

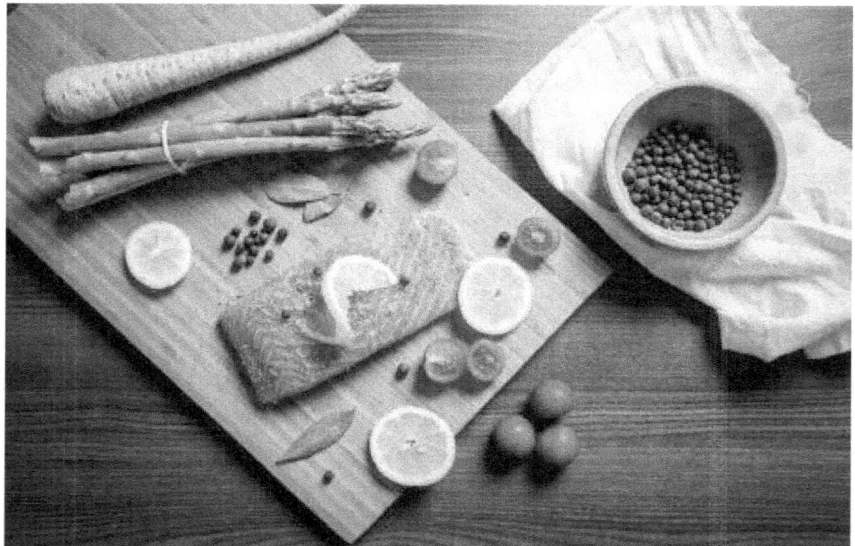

HOW ANTI INFLAMMATORY DIET WORKS

Inflammation has always been a therapeutic secret, yet now it has turned into a foe of long haul health. From one perspective, when your skin turns red, swollen, and painful after you consume yourself, which triggers intense inflammation, the reaction is ordinary and advantageous. Additional red platelets, safe cells, and antioxidants are hurrying to the injured site to recuperate it. In any case, conveyed excessively thus far, inflammation can be lethal, as when somebody is too scorched to even consider recovering.

Just in a couple that is previous of, has it unfolded that low-level incessant inflammation, which ordinarily goes unnoticed, has an influence on numerous life disorders, for example, hypertension, heart disease, cancer, and Alzheimer's disease. Synthetic compounds known as inflammation markers can enter the circulatory system in different ways: from the intestinal tract (purported flawed gut), as a response to disease, or through the activity of the safe framework in other inward ways. The moderate trickle, dribble of inflammatory markers, can take a very long time to make real impedance, which implies that every individual must tailor his way of life to counter them. Diet alone is not sufficient to keep ceaseless, intense inflammation under control...yet it is a decent start. The Mediterranean diet has been known to help lessen inflammation in the body, so it is an incredible way to kick-start your diet. By embracing an anti-inflammatory diet, you go for two positive outcomes: keeping the microorganisms in your digestive tracts healthy and flourishing, thereby avoiding the drainage of lethal synthetics into the circulation system. There is additionally the circuitous benefit that a healthy stomach related framework, sends a sign of prosperity along the vagus nerve to the heart and cerebrum. There is a huge number of microorganisms that possess the intestinal tract, and are a fundamental piece of our complete DNA, contributing a great many separate genomes. Together this tremendous settlement is known as the microbiome. Here are some basic focuses to know. The gut microbiome is not the same as a culture to culture. In every one of us, it is always moves accordingly to the diet, yet to pressure and even feelings. Because of its hereditary, multifaceted nature, an "ordinary" gut microbiome has not been characterized at this point. It is accepted that flourishing, healthy gut microbiome is established on a wide scope of common foods wealthy in fruits, vegetables, and fiber. The cutting edge Western diet, which is low in fiber, yet high in sugar, salt, fat, and handling food, might be genuinely debasing the gut microbiome. At the point when the gut microbiome is harmed or debased, microscopic organisms start to discharge supposed endotoxins—the results of microbial activity. If these poisons spill through the intestinal divider into the circulatory system, markers for inflammation are activated, and persevere until the poisons are never again present.

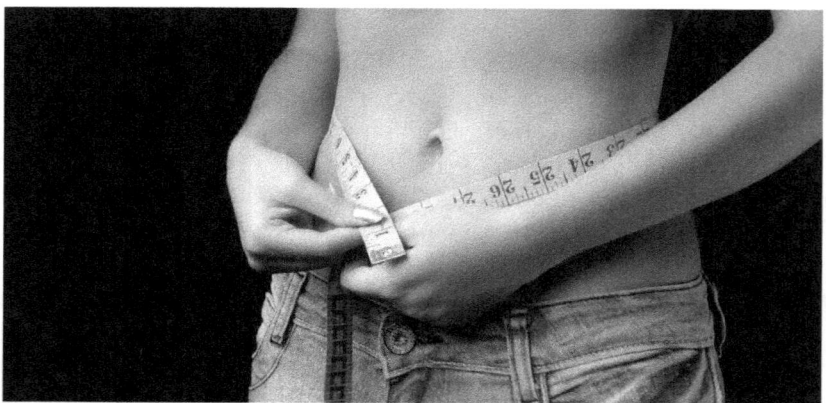

WHAT IS INFLAMMATION?

Inflammation is the body's reaction to diseases, including contaminations or wounds. The immune system sends an increased measure of white blood cells to the region fending off the disease or destroy. Inflammation is not generally a terrible thing; it is only the body attempting to shield itself from further damage or disease by expanding the immune reaction in the region being compromised by microbes or damage. Nonetheless, there are a few incessant inflammatory diseases. For example, joint pain, psoriasis, and asthma that can make the immune system go into overdrive and assault solid tissues. Inflammation is a characteristic procedure with the organic reason to start mending by expanding course. It is a mind-boggling procedure, including both the immune system and vascular system, and the exchange of different concoction go-betweens. The increased course brings white blood cells and sustenance to the site of damage or disease with the goal that attacking pathogens are slaughtered, and harm might be fixed. Trademark indications of inflammation incorporate pain (dolor), heat, swelling (tumor), and redness (rubor). As a feature of the inflammatory reaction, your body increases its creation of white blood cells, immune cells, and substances called cytokines that help battle disease.

Great indications of acute (present moment) inflammation incorporate: redness, pain, warmth, and swelling. On the other hand, unending (long haul) inflammation frequently happens inside your body, with no perceptible manifestations. This sort of inflammation can drive sicknesses like diabetes, heart disease, greasy liver disease, and cancer.

SIDE EFFECTS OF INFLAMMATION

Side effects of inflammation differ, and are contingent upon whether the response is acute or incessant. The impacts of acute inflammation can be summed up below:

- **Pain:** The aggravated region is probably going to be painful, particularly during and in the wake of contact. Synthetic substances that invigorate nerve endings are discharged, making the region increasingly touchy.
- **Redness:** This occurs because the vessels in the zone are loaded up with more blood than expected.
- **Immobility:** There might be some loss of capacity in the area of the inflammation.
- **Swelling:** This is brought about by the development of liquid.
- **Heat**: More bloodstreams to the influenced territory, making it feel warm to the touch.

These acute inflammation signs and symptoms apply to inflammations of the skin. On the off chance that inflammation happens somewhere inside the body, for example, in an inward organ, just a portion of the signs might be perceptible. For instance, some interior organs might not have tactile nerve endings adjacent, so there will be no pain. This may include particular kinds of lung inflammation. Side effects of interminable inflammation may present in an alternate manner. These can incorporate exhaustion, mouth injuries, chest pain, stomach pain, fever, rash, joint pain, and so on.

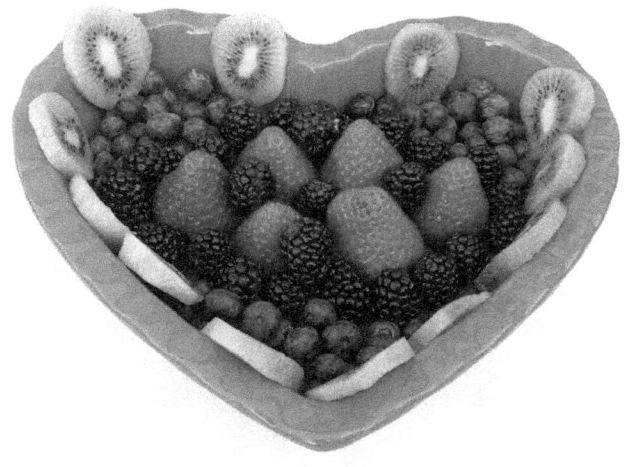

WHY EXCESSIVE INFLAMMATION IS SO COMMON

On the off chance that inflammation is a characteristic and important piece of the body's guards, what is causing this well-planned framework to breakdown? For what reason are such a significant number of us experiencing intemperate inflammation? The appropriate response is unpredictable, yet it comes down to this: *we have lost our equalization*. The body's inflammation reaction works through two reciprocal channels: one is professional inflammatory and the other anti-inflammatory. Our phones produce an assortment of star and anti-inflammatory synthetic substances (called prostaglandins), utilizing supplements from the sustenance we eat as the crude material.

These prostaglandins are discharged into our tissues in light of the invulnerable framework's sign, advancing inflammation when there is a risk and suppressing inflammation when the threat has passed. A key idea in this (misrepresented) depiction is that our bodies produce prostaglandins by utilizing mixes from the sustenance we eat. In particular, it is the unsaturated fats in our nourishments, that our bodies use to make prostaglandins. Particular kinds of unsaturated fats (principally those from the omega-6 family) are changed over into inflammatory prostaglandins, while different sorts are utilized to make anti-inflammatory prostaglandins. This is the place we, as a cutting edge society, have fallen into difficulty. To keep up a harmony between its star and anti-inflammatory channels, the body depends on a reasonable admission of omega-3 and omega-6 unsaturated fats. The issue is that those of us who live in current modern countries devour awfully numerous omega-6 unsaturated fats and extremely couple of omega-3 unsaturated fats. Scientists and anthropologists gauge that the diet of a Stone Age human contained generally a balance of omega-3 and omega-6 unsaturated fats. Today, we devour around twenty fold the amount of omega-6 as we do omega-3. Accordingly, our bodies will, in general, produce an excess of genius inflammatory prostaglandins, and a lack of anti-inflammatory prostaglandins. The Inflammation-Free Diet restores a characteristic equalization and turns around this risky pattern.

INFLAMMATION: WHO IS AT RISK?

For all intents and purposes, any individual who eats a cutting edge. The western diet is at risk of inordinate inflammation, for the reasons simply given. However, there are different factors that can expand the affinity toward inflammation or inflammation-related disease:

• **Smoking**: Smoking makes colossal quantities of free radicals, which thus produce inflammation in the tissues. Particularly influenced are the cells coating the bronchial entries and the little veins that lead to the heart. Smokers more often than not have abnormal amounts of inflammatory synthetic concoctions in their blood, and a significantly expanded risk of numerous inflammation-related diseases.

• **Excess weight**: Adults and youngsters who are overweight likewise will, in general, have larger amounts of inflammatory synthetic concoctions in their blood than those of ordinary weight. This is aggravated by the way that the individuals who are overweight will, in general, be less dynamic...which further adds to inflammation.

• **Sedentary Way of Life**: Among its numerous advantages, practice will balance the body's expert and anti-inflammatory channels—gave, obviously, that no wounds are supported! Exercise additionally, aids in decreasing inflammation by moderating the impacts of pressure.

• **Stress**: Chronic pressure (Common) an excessive number of requests insufficient time sort—significantly adjusts our interior science in manners that add to inflammation. Adrenaline and cortisol, the supposed pressure hormones, drain our supply of DHEA (a hormone that is a characteristic anti-inflammatory specialist).

• **Unprotected Sun Presentation**: The sun's bright beams make free radicals and inflammation when they strike unprotected skin. This inflammatory procedure in the skin is accepted to be an essential factor in the improvement of lines, wrinkles, age spots, and skin malignant growth.

• **Hormone Substitution Treatment**: Studies have discovered that generally sound ladies taking hormone substitution prescriptions, have fundamentally increased inflammatory synthetics in their blood than ladies who do not utilize hormones. This might be a contributing factor in the expanded risk of heart disease and malignant growth in ladies utilizing hormone substitution.

• **Disease**: Degenerative diseases (for example, heart disease, Alzheimer's disease, malignant growth, diabetes, rheumatoid joint pain, lupus, and numerous sclerosis) advance inordinate inflammation in the body. You may have side effects, such as those recorded in the list below, which makes it clear inflammation, is an issue for you. On the other hand, maybe at least one of the inflammation risk factors just talked about (smoking or being overweight) concerns you. Frequently, be that as it may, fundamental inflammation does not deliver any indications or cautioning signs.

> - Allergies.
> - Premature skin maturing.
> - Prostatitis.
> - Skin issue and so forth.

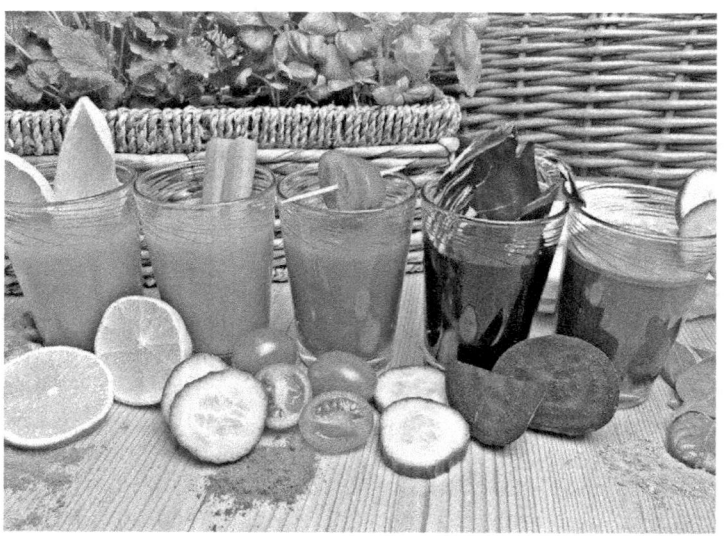

IT CAN HARM YOUR GUT

A large number of the body's immune cells bunch around the digestive organs. More often than not, those immune cells disregard the trillions of solid microorganisms that live in the gut. "Be that as it may, for certain people, that resistance is by all accounts broken, and their immune cells begin to respond to the microbes, making interminable inflammation. The immune cells can assault the stomach related tract itself, an autoimmune condition known as inflammatory bowel disease (IBD), which incorporates ulcerative colitis and Crohn's disease. The indications incorporate loose bowels, spasms, ulcers, and may even require careful expulsion of the digestive organs. Specialists are not actually certain why a few people get IBD, yet hereditary qualities, condition, anti-infection agents, diet, and stress the board all appear to assume a job.

At the point when inflammation happens in the joints, it can cause genuine harm. One joint-harming condition is Rheumatoid joint pain (RA), another case of an autoimmune issue that seems to have a hereditary part, but at the same time, is connected to smoking, an absence of nutrient D, and other risk factors. Studies found that a salty eating regimen may add to the advancement of RA. People with RA experience pain and firmness in their aggravated joints. However, since the immune response is not constrained to the joints, they are likewise at a higher risk for issues with their eyes and other body parts. Psoriatic joint inflammation additionally includes inflammation in the joints, and its indications are like those of RA. In any case, notwithstanding painful, firm joints, people with PsA may likewise experience changes in the nails, such as setting. A great many people with psoriatic joint pain initially create psoriasis, another autoimmune condition, on their skin. Around 30% of people with psoriasis are thought to create psoriatic joint pain, and you might be bound to do as such if your skin psoriasis influences your nails.

LINKED TO HEART DISEASE

Any piece of your body that has been harmed or will be harmed can trigger inflammation, even the inner parts of blood vessels. The arrangement of greasy plaque in the corridors can trigger unending inflammation. The greasy plaques draw in white blood cells, become bigger, and can frame blood clumps, which can cause a heart assault. One explicit protein, called interleukin-6 (IL-6), may assume a key job, as indicated by a 2012 study distributed in The Lancet. Heftiness and undesirable eating increase inflammation in the body, yet even generally solid people who experience incessant inflammation on account of an autoimmune issue (rheumatoid joint pain, psoriasis, or celiac disease) seem to have a higher risk of heart disease, paying little respect to their weight or dietary patterns.

HIGHER RISK OF CANCER

Unending inflammation has been connected to cancers of the lung, throat, cervix, and stomach related tract, among others. A 2014 Harvard University study found that large young people with abnormal amounts of inflammation had a 63% increased risk of creating colorectal cancer during adulthood, contrasted with their more slender friends. The inflammation might be because of stoutness, interminable contamination, a synthetic aggravation, or perpetual condition; all have been connected to higher cancer risk. At the point when immune cells begin to deliver inflammation, immune guideline moves toward becoming disintegrated, and it makes an operation disrupt your rest. People who announced dozing more than normal had more elevated amounts of inflammation-related proteins in their blood than the individuals who said they dozed about 7.6 hours a night. This exploration just settled a connection between the two (and not circumstances and logical results), so the study creators state they cannot make certain whether inflammation triggers, long and short rest term or whether rest span triggers inflammation. It is additionally conceivable that an alternate basic issue, as constant pressure or disease, causes both. More work has likewise been found to increase inflammation in the body.

IT'S BAD FOR YOUR LUNGS

At the point when inflammation happens in the lungs, it can cause liquid amassing and narrowing of the aviation routes, making it hard to relax. Contaminations, asthma, and Ceaseless Obstructive Pneumonic Disease (COPD - which incorporates emphysema and perpetual bronchitis) are altogether portrayed by inflammation in the lungs. Smoking, introduction of air contamination or family synthetic substances, being overweight, and even utilization of restored meats, have been connected to lung inflammation.

IT DAMAGES GUMS

Inflammation can likewise unleash destruction on your mouth as periodontitis, an unending inflammation of the gums brought about by microorganisms gathering. This disease makes gums subside, and the skeletal structure around the teeth become debilitated or harmed. Brushing and flossing normally can anticipate periodontitis, and one 2010 Harvard University study found that eating calming omega-3 unsaturated fats (for example fish or fish oil) may likewise help. Periodontal disease does not simply influence oral wellbeing, either. Studies demonstrate that inflammation of the gums is connected to heart disease and dementia, too; since microscopic organisms in the mouth may likewise trigger inflammation somewhere else in the body.

IT MAKES WEIGHT LOSS MORE DIFFICULT

Heftiness is a noteworthy reason for inflammation in the body, and getting more fit is one of the best approaches to battle it. In some cases, more difficult than one might expect, because raised degrees of inflammation-related proteins can likewise make weight loss more troublesome than it ought to be. First, perpetual inflammation can influence hunger signals and hinder digestion, so you eat more and burn fewer calories. Inflammation can likewise increase insulin resistance (which raises your risk for diabetes) and has been connected with future weight gain. It makes weight loss increasingly troublesome. Stoutness is a noteworthy reason for inflammation in the body, and shedding pounds is one of the best approaches to battle it. In any case, that is sometimes actually quite difficult, because raised degrees of inflammation-related proteins can likewise make weight loss more troublesome than it ought to be. First off, unending inflammation can influence hunger signals and hinder digestion, so you eat more and burn fewer calories. Inflammation can likewise increase insulin resistance (which raises your risk for diabetes) and has been connected with future weight gain. Inflammation of the gastrointestinal tract (similarly as with inflammatory bowel disease) can be particularly adverse to bone wellbeing, since it can avert retention of significant bone-building supplements for example, calcium and nutrient D. Another inflammatory disease, rheumatoid joint pain, can likewise have suggestions since it confines people's physical movement and can shield them from performing weight-bearing, bone-reinforcing works out.

IT AFFECTS YOUR SKIN

The impacts of inflammation are not simple, but can also be contributed to your skin. Psoriasis, for instance. Psoriasis is a common skin condition that speeds up the life cycle of skin cells. It causes cells to build up rapidly on the surface of the skin. The extra skin cells form scales and red patches that are itchy and sometimes painful.

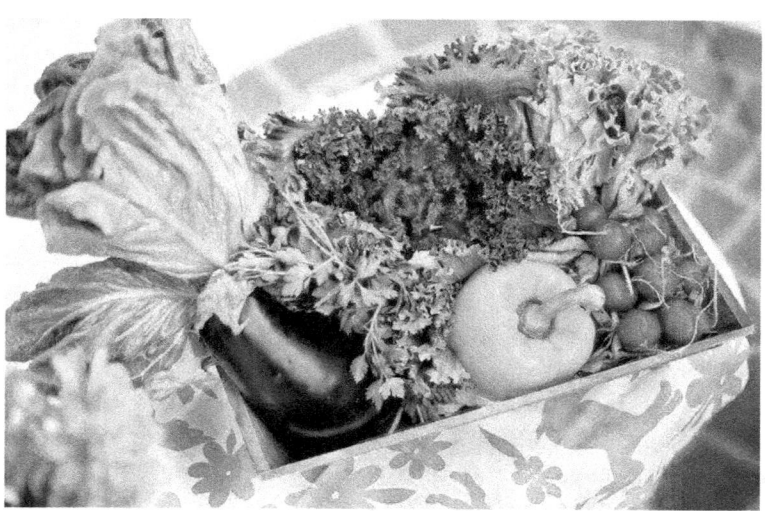

ANTI-INFLAMMATORY DIET: SAMPLE MEAL PLAN

Breakfast

- Coconut Milk, Old Fashioned Oats or cracked grain cereal
- Chia seeds
- Ground flax seeds
- Nuts or other seeds
- Cinnamon

Lunch

- Spinach, kale, romaine, etc.
- Carrots, broccoli, tomato, peppers, purple onion, avocado
- Chicken or seafood of choice
- Soy nuts, or other types of nut or seeds
- Fresh Fruit

Dinner

- Salmon/other seafood or lean meat
- Sweet potato or squash
- Broccoli
- Salad greens with chopped vegetables
- Fruit

Snack

- 6 whole almonds or other nuts
- Apple or other fruit

ANTI-INFLAMMATORY DIETS: RULES FOR OPTIMAL HEALTH

Lowering inflammation is crucial if you are aiming at long-term good health. Inflammation is the body causes or contributes to many debilitating and chronic illnesses like rheumatoid arthritis, heart disease, Alzheimer's disease, and cancer. Physicians and nutritionists I recommend patients to eat a diet focused on anti-inflammatory principles. Recent research discovered that eating this diet slows the ageing process by stabilizing blood sugar and increasing metabolism

- Consume between 20 - 50 grams of fiber each day.
- Sweeten your meals with phytonutrient-rich fruits, and flavor foods with spices.
- Avoid processed foods and refined sugars.
- Eat a minimum of eight servings of vegetables daily.
- Eat four servings of alliums and crucifers weekly.
- Cut back saturated fat to 10 percent of your daily calories.
- Eat fish at least three times weekly.
- Go for both low-fat fish such as sole and flounder and cold-water fish that contain healthy fats.
- Use oils that contain healthy fats.
- Eat healthy snacks twice a day.
- Eat five to nine servings of antioxidant-rich foods grown from the ground each day.
- Replace red meat with more advantageous protein sources, such as lean poultry, fish, soy, beans, and lentils.
- Avoid margarine and vegetable oils and go for more advantageous fats found in olive oil, nuts, and seeds.
- Instead of choosing refined grains, decide on fiber-rich entire grains like oats, quinoa, dark colored rice, bread, and pasta that rundown an entire grain as the primary fixing.
- Rather than flavoring your suppers with salt, enhance with anti-inflammatory herbs like garlic, ginger, and turmeric.

ADVANTAGES OF ANTI INFLAMMATORY DIETS

In spite of the fact that weight reduction is the essential objective of most dietary examples, the focal point of an anti-inflammatory diet is on controlling wellbeing conditions. Indeed, even the individuals who do not experience the ill effects of any chronic disease may profit by reducing their risk of creating one. This is achieved by choosing and maintaining a strategic distance from foods to reduce inflammation in the body. Notwithstanding, it is significant that there are two sorts of inflammation. Acute inflammation is an ordinary reaction in our body, which occurs directly after damage or ailment. While it plays out a helpful function in these scenarios by shielding the body, the reaction can be unsafe in the event that it occurs over a drawn-out period — this is known as chronic inflammation.

As wellbeing research has proposed, chronic inflammation may contribute to the improvement of a few diseases, including lupus, cancer, stroke, and the sky is the limit from there. Similarly, as with all nourishment rules, an abundance of leafy foods is encouraged in this diet. In particular, include increasingly green verdant vegetables, tomatoes, and natural products like strawberries, blueberries, and oranges. Rather than meat, decide on eating fish twice per week to get your required portion of omega-3 fats.

Anti-inflammatory food components protect the body against the conceivable harm caused by inflammation. The diet additionally has a decent amount of flavor — certain spices like garlic and turmeric have been connected to anti-inflammatory properties. With some restraint, one can likewise appreciate coffee, nuts and seeds, dim chocolate, etc. for comparable properties. With respect to foods to exclude, avoid processed meat, vegetable oils, sugary refreshments like soft drinks, and refined carbohydrates like white bread. Overwhelming drinking has additionally been connected to inflammation, so make a point to direct your alcohol admission.

Dairy seems to remain on the fence between anti-inflammatory and expert inflammatory. Researchers note that it, to a great extent, relies upon the individual and how tolerant their body is when processing lactose. Therefore, it might look for advice from a dietitian and watch your own flare-ups to recognize what sort of dairy you ought to settle on. Irrespective of the fact that it is anything but a cure, this diet may help any individual who experiences a condition associated with inflammation. Physicians recommend this eating design for rheumatoid joint pain patients. Many have likewise thought about whether inflammation is more about quantity than quality, for example, in the event that the calorie admission is to be faulted instead of the kind of food we consume. In any case, research has discovered that the connection exists notwithstanding when stoutness and weight increase are accounted for. A portion of the food components or fixings may effectively affect inflammation far beyond increased caloric admission. A portion of the advantages of the anti-inflammatory diet include:

YOU FEEL MORE ENERGIZED

An anti-inflammatory diet exhorts constraining excess sugar and embracing sound entire grains—two changes which can be proven to increase vitality levels. That is because sugar gives you an instant shock pursued by an inescapable crash (like the manner in which you feel a few hours after that morning croissant and sweetened coffee). However, entire grains are assimilated much slower in the human body, giving you a drawn-out vitality discharge. Take a stab at kicking off your morning with one of these medium-term oat recipes in place of your standard breakfast request.

YOU MIGHT LOSE SOME WEIGHT

While the primary objective of an AI eating plan is not to shed pounds, numerous individuals who attempt it report weight reduction as a common symptom. A five-year concentrate distributed in The Lancet Diabetes and Endocrinology found that individuals who pursued an anti-inflammatory Mediterranean diet lost more weight than the individuals who went on a low-fat arrangement. Also, according to another investigation by Tufts University, entire grains could accelerate your digestion—participants with a diet rich in entire grains (like entire grain bread) lost a normal of 100 calories more for every day than those eating refined carbohydrates (like white rice).

YOU MAY FEEL HAPPIER

The Mediterranean diet could actually help your mind-set. In the examination, scientists checked a gathering of individuals with melancholy for 12 weeks as they pursued the anti-inflammatory diet, and the lion's share announced a major improvement of their side effects.

YOU MAY HAVE LESS JOINT PAIN REDUCE YOUR RISK OF BONE LOSS

An anti-inflammatory diet could improve joint wellbeing and help reduce a portion of the excruciating manifestations of joint inflammation. Despite the fact that there is no diet cure for joint inflammation, certain foods have been appeared to battle inflammation, fortify bones, and lift the insusceptible framework. The research found that ladies with diets that are low in inflammatory foods lost less bone thickness in a six-year time span than those that included progressively inflammatory foods (despite the fact that the less inflammatory gathering had a lower bone thickness in any case). The investigation likewise found that the diet was connected to fewer hip fractures.

HINDERED COGNITIVE AGING

Antioxidant-rich berries are probably the best anti-inflammatory foods around, and information from one long haul concentrate distributed in the field of nervous system science found that they may postpone cognitive maturing. Utilizing memory and thinking tests, researchers discovered that a higher admission of berries reduces paces of cognitive decline in old ladies by as much as over two years. Berries, with the largest amounts of flavonoids, such as blueberries and strawberries, had the most advantage, according to researchers. They are additionally the most delicious.

LIFT YOUR HEART HEALTH

To recap, the anti-inflammatory Mediterranean diet is actually damn extraordinary for you. Be that as it may, conceivably the greatest advantageous asset of all? It reduces the possibility of coronary illness. Sticking with the food diet might be going to reduce your levels of low-thickness lipoprotein (LDL) cholesterol, otherwise referred to as "awful" type of cholesterol that may develop stores in your supply routes.

TOP INFLAMMATION CURING FOOD

Inflammation is your insusceptible framework's reaction to aggravation, damage, or infection. It is an ordinary reaction (and actually something to be thankful for), and it is a characteristic piece of mending. In any case, it is conceivable that chronic inflammation could negatively affect your body and your wellbeing. Following an anti-inflammatory diet is one approach to counter a portion of the chronic inflammation that comes from driving a not really solid way of life. In case you are prepared to get back on the way to smart dieting, attempt these foods that are for the most part nutritious and fit perfectly into an anti-inflammatory diet.

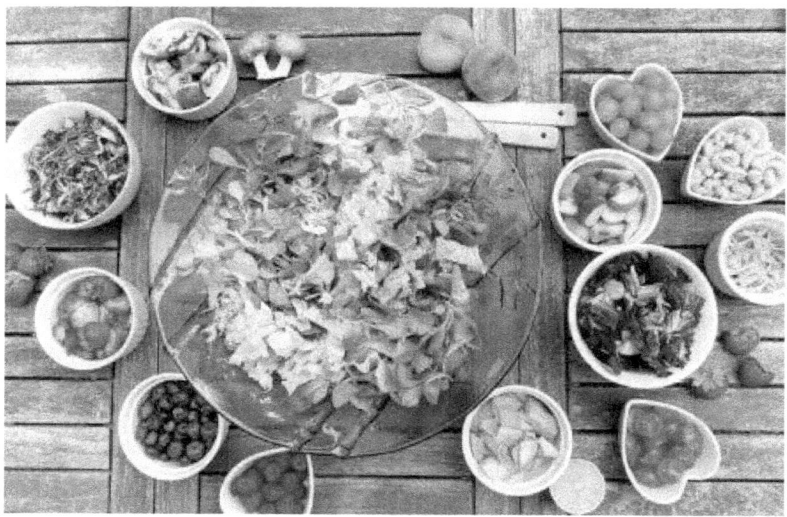

ALMONDS

They are an overwhelming source of unsaturated fats, vitamin E, and manganese. They are likewise a decent source of magnesium and plant protein. In research thinks about, eating almonds has been associated with having a lower risk of cardiovascular disease, likely by improving the fatty acids profile of your blood. Almonds are likewise very satisfying, so despite the fact that they are somewhat higher in calories than numerous other anti-inflammatory foods, eating a bunch of almonds may enable you to stick with a solid health improvement plan.

AVOCADOS

Avocados are rich in heart-solid monounsaturated fats. Eating a large portion of avocado will likewise add nicely to your day-by-day admission of vitamins C, And, E, and B-complex vitamins. The combination of these supplements and the polyphenols that work as antioxidants make avocados an absolute necessity have for any anti-inflammatory diet. Add avocado slices to your preferred sandwich or serving of mixed greens, or make scrumptious guacamole.

FATTY FISH

Fatty fish are an incredible source of protein and the long-chain omega-3 fatty acids EPA and DHA. Albeit a wide range of fish contain some omega-3 fatty acids, these fatty fish are among the best sources are Salmon , Sardines, Herring, Mackerel, Anchovies, EPA and DHA reduce inflammation that can prompt metabolic disorder, coronary illness, diabetes and kidney diseases.

PEPPERS

Chime peppers and chili peppers are stacked with vitamin C and antioxidants that have amazing anti-inflammatory effects. Chime peppers give the antioxidant quercetin, which may reduce one marker of oxidative harm in individuals.

BROCCOLI

Broccoli is an individual from the cruciferous group of vegetables that are high in phytochemicals called glucosinolates. These phytochemicals are amazing antioxidants. Broccoli is likewise an excellent source of vitamin C, potassium, calcium, and vitamin A, all while being low in calories. It is anything but difficult to get more broccoli into your diet because it is delicious cooked or crude. Epidemiological investigations demonstrate that eating a diet high in cruciferous vegetables, including broccoli, is associated with having a lower risk of certain kinds of cancer.

OLIVE OIL

Olive oil is a component of the anti-inflammatory eating regimen, which has been linked to heart wellbeing and life span. It's rich in polyphenols that work as antioxidants to protect the cells in your body. Olive oil reduces irritation, reduces elevated cholesterol, and it's possible that a portion of the polyphenols may help counteract a few types of cancer, so it's an astounding oil to add to your Kitchen.

DRY BEANS

Dry beans, for instance, navy beans, kidney beans, pinto beans, and black beans, are an extraordinary calming source of plant protein, minerals, B-complex vitamins, and vitamin K. They're furthermore chock-brimming with useful fibre, and also contain polyphenols that work as antioxidants.

MUSHROOM

While a large number of assortments of mushrooms exist around the world, just a couple are edible and developed financially. These incorporate truffles, portobello mushrooms, and shiitake. Mushrooms are low in calories and wealthy in selenium, copper, and the entirety of the B vitamins. They likewise contain phenols and different antioxidants that give anti-inflammatory protection.

GRAPES

Grapes contain anthocyanins, which reduce inflammation. Likewise, they may decrease the danger of several diseases, including heart disease, diabetes, obesity, Alzheimer's disease, and eye disorders. Grapes are likewise one of the best sources of resveratrol, and also aggravate that has numerous health benefits.

WALNUT

Walnuts are a good source of fats, protein, vitamin E, minerals, and phytochemicals called sterols. They likewise contain monounsaturated

unsaturated fats and omega-3 unsaturated fats that are useful for your heart. Walnuts are likewise energy-dense, so you may need to watch your bit size, yet even however they are high in calories, eating a bunch of walnuts can help you feel full longer and really help you lose weight.

SWISS CHARD

Swiss chard is so beautiful and delicious. It's a wonderful (and brilliant) leafy vegetable to add to your anti-inflammatory shopping list. It's an excellent source of vitamins A and K, a good source of numerous minerals and very low in calories.

SWEET POTATOES

They are amazingly rich in vitamins and minerals; they are amazingly high in vitamin A and beta-carotene, which is a powerful antioxidant. Sweet potatoes likewise are an excellent source of numerous vitamins and minerals, including vitamins C and K, potassium, and B complex vitamins. Sweet potatoes additionally have a lot of fibre and aren't excessively high in calories, so they make a delicious option to any diet.

SPINACH

Spinach is a standout amongst another known of all the anti-inflammatory superfoods. It contains lutein, which is identified with vitamin A and beta-carotene. Spinach additionally gives you iron, vitamin K, and folate, and it is low in calories, so it's perfect for weight loss diets. Research shows that individuals who eat green, verdant vegetables, like spinach, may have a decreased risk of macular degeneration, so include a lot of new or cooked spinach to your diet.

STRAWBERRIES

Strawberries are delicious, juicy, and sweet, and they're also good for your health. It is very low in calories, high in fibre, and they contain vitamins and minerals your body needs to function properly, including a lot of vitamin C. They also have anti-inflammatory properties and lots of potential health advantages.

DARK CHOCOLATE

Make the most of your treat! Dark chocolate with at any rate 70% cocoa is rich in flavanols, which may lower pulse. Eat dark chocolate with some restraint as it is additionally overflowing with calories – two ounces packs around 300 calories. Spot a bit of dark chocolate on your tongue, close your eyes, and enjoy it. You'll see that you just need a modest quantity to fulfill your taste buds.

CORE VALUE TO CHOOSING A MEAL PLAN

Concentrate on a plant-based eating routine

Prepared foods, in addition to dairy, sugar, and bread, can be delectable, but at the same time, they're ace inflammatory. Adhering to gluten-free side-dishes like buckwheat, quinoa, amaranth, and cauliflower 'rice' are great substitutes for prepared carbs, and sub in agave or date syrup or modest quantities of maple syrup for sugar. To be perfectly honest, as a veggie-lover, I accept dairy and meat ought to be off the menu by and large, however on the off chance that you should, guarantee these are natural, at least. Feel free to go insane on the accompanying foods, which are tops for reducing inflammation:

- celery, verdant greens, broccoli, beets, bok choi, garlic, onions.
- fruits like pineapple, red grapes, berries, or acai.
- walnuts, coconut oil, olive oil, chia seed, flaxseed.
- ginger, turmeric, cinnamon, green tea.

Heap on the Omegas

Fat is great. A few fats, in any event, to be specific Omega-3 and -6 fats, at the point when consolidated in the correct ways, these two can truly lessen inflammation keep every one of your cells working ideally. Disregard bringing down enhancements – the ideal approach to get these is straightforwardly from food. Think pecans, flaxseed, chia seeds, mung beans, and hemp oil frequently.

Chill Out

One of the significant reasons for inflammation is stress. It expedites it, on account of the genius inflammatory impacts of constantly raised cortisol levels, which increment the generation of inflammatory cytokines. So the sooner you begin relaxing, the better. All your dedicated eating routine endeavours will be futile in the event that you don't reflect, take full breaths when you're feeling pushed, go on more occasions, or simply maintain a strategic distance from pressure at whatever point possible. Some of the recipes incorporate.

BENEFITS OF REDUCING INFLAMMATION

The Inflammation-Free Diet will help to rebalance the pro- and anti-inflammatory channels in your body and reduce excessive inflammation. If you currently have symptoms related to inflammation, such as joint pain, hay fever, asthma, or skin allergies, you will most likely notice a substantial improvement in these symptoms within a few weeks. The Inflammation-Free Diet will also help rejuvenate your skin, smoothing fine lines and wrinkles and improving your skin's texture and clarity. In addition to these immediate benefits, isn't it wonderful to know that by reducing inflammation, you are also lowering your chances of serious disease in the future like heart diseases, Alzheimer and cancer amongothers.

TOWARDS A BETTER INFLAMMATORY LIFESTYLE

Inflammation is one of the body's normal methods for ensuring itself. It includes numerous concoction responses that help to fend off contaminations, increment bloodstream to places that need mending and produce torment as a sign that something isn't right with the body. Lamentably, similarly, as with any procedure in the body, it is conceivable to have an overdose of something that is otherwise good. Inflammation is regularly contrasted with flame. In controlled sums, there is no doubt that fire keeps us warm, solid, and secured, however when there is a lot of flames, or if fire gains out of power, it very well may be ruinous. Be that as it may, a flame shouldn't be huge to cause harm. It is currently comprehended that poor quality perpetual or on-going inflammation that is underneath the degree of agony can add to numerous ceaseless medical issues and would itself be able to turn into a sickness. This poor quality inflammation can keep the body's tissues from appropriately fixing and furthermore start to crush sound cells in supply routes, organs, joints, and different parts of the body. How we eat can influence inflammation, and certain diets are bound to diminish torment and different side effects of sickness. It is assessed that 60% of interminable infections, including a considerable lot of the medical issues recorded above, could be anticipated by a solid diet. Not exclusively can eating the correct sustenance decrease the event of inflammation in any case. However, it can likewise diminish and resolve inflammation that is as of now happening. Eating to diminish inflammation isn't one-size-fits-all. Various individuals will do it in various ways. One of the most examined instances of a mitigating method for eating is the conventional Mediterranean diet, which is a dietary example propelled by certain nations of the Mediterranean bowl. Individuals that all the more intently eat a Mediterranean-like diet has reliably lower levels of inflammation contrasted with different fewer sound methods for eating. The Mediterranean diet has been broadly examined and is defensive against numerous perpetual wellbeing conditions including cardiovascular illness, type 2 diabetes mellitus, Parkinson's and Alzheimer's sickness, and a few tumours. The Mediterranean diet is only one case of a customary diet and happens to be the most inquired about conventional diet design on the planet. Numerous customary diets are more beneficial than in vogue present-day diets since they are revolved around eating entire, natural sustenance's, imparted to loved ones. The points of interest of the Mediterranean Diet may change from concentrate to contemplate, yet these are constantly normal components. You can control and even turn around inflammation through a sound, calming way of life. Individuals with a family ancestry of medical issues, for example, coronary illness or colon malignant growth, should converse with their doctors about the way of life changes that help to avoid sickness by decreasing inflammation. Follow these tips for reducing inflammation in your body:

Load up on anti-inflammatory foods

Your food decisions are similarly as significant as the meds and enhancements you might take for generally speaking wellbeing since they can secure against inflammation. An anti-inflammatory diet accentuates foods that reduce inflammation, Eat more products of the soil, and foods containing omega-3 unsaturated fats. The absolute best sources of omega-3s are virus water fish, for example, salmon and fish, and tofu, pecans, flax seeds, and soybeans. Other anti-inflammatory foods incorporate grapes, celery, blueberries, garlic, olive oil, tea, and a few flavors (ginger, rosemary, and turmeric). The Mediterranean diet is a case of an anti-inflammatory diet. This is because of its emphasis on organic products, vegetables, fish and entire grains, and points of confinement on undesirable fats, for example, red meat, margarine, and egg yolks just as processed and refined sugars and carbs.

Cut back or take out inflammatory foods

An anti-inflammatory diet additionally confines foods that advance inflammation; inflammatory foods incorporate red meat and anything with Tran's fats, for example, margarine, corn oil, pan-fried foods, and most processed foods.

Control glucose

Cutoff or dodge straightforward starches, for example, white flour, white rice, refined sugar, and anything with high fructose corn syrup. One simple standard to pursue is to keep away from white foods, for example, white bread, rice, and pasta, just as foods made with white sugar and flour. Fabricate dinners around lean proteins and entire foods high in fibre, for example, vegetables, products of the soil grains, for example, dark colored rice and entire wheat bread. Check the marks and ensure that "entire wheat" or another entire grain is the principal ingredient.

Set aside a few minutes to exercise

Customary exercise is a great method to avoid inflammation, Make time for 30 to 45 minutes of high-impact exercise, and 10 to 25 minutes of weight or obstruction preparing, in any event, four to five times each week. Individuals who are overweight have more inflammation. Shedding pounds may diminish inflammation.

Control Red Meat Intake

Individuals that eat the absolute red meat stay at most serious hazard for diabetes, cardiovascular illness, and various diseases. Notwithstanding, late proof recommends that processed red meats, like hot dogs, frankfurter, and lunch meats, might be the greatest offender.

Red meat is a decent source of protein, iron, and different micronutrients. However, poultry, eggs, and dairy just as plant proteins (vegetables), and grains can fill in as great substitutes. In the event that you expend red meat, select grass-bolstered unprocessed sources that may have progressively positive unsaturated fat profiles, pick lean cuts and cut back obvious excess. The World Cancer Research Fund proposes eating close to 12 to 18 ounces, cooked weight, of red meat every week (three 6oz servings or six 3oz servings); 3oz is about the size of a deck of cards. Stay away from processed meats, for example, ham, salami, hot dogs, and hotdogs.

Moderate Dairy Intake

Full-fat and non-matured dairy may barely affect expanding inflammation, however by and large, dairy does not appear to build inflammation. Besides, aged dairy like yoghurt and Kiefer have an impartial or even constructive outcome on both cardiovascular hazard and inflammation. Therefore utilization of dairy, and particularly yoghurt in moderate sums, might be a satisfactory piece of an anti-inflammatory method for eating. Make certain to confine sugar intake by picking plain, unsweetened assortments.

Eat Low-Glycemic Load (GL)

Eat low GL foods and dinner designs. These foods incorporate complex sugars (for example, unprocessed entire grains, bland vegetables, and natural products), protein, fats, and foods rich in fibre that help to keep glucose stable and reduce the inflammatory effects of insulin. By devouring complex starches in the mix with foods that are high in fibre and sound oils, sugar separate is eased back, and the general glycemic load is reduced.

Eat more fibre

Fibre eases back the absorption of starches, directing glucose levels, and likewise keeping you full more. Instruments by which fibre reduces inflammation are not so much seen. However, fibre energizes reusing of fats in the body and furthermore supports great microorganisms in the digestive organs that decidedly influence inflammatory pathways. Likewise, entire foods rich in fibre contain other significant phytochemicals that have anti-inflammatory effects.

Ensure Adequate Magnesium (Mg) Intake

Mg deficiency is connected to increased inflammation. Mg is under-devoured in the US due to poor diet, and it is assessed that 60% of Americans don't get enough.34 Dark verdant vegetables are a rich source of Mg just as vegetables, nuts, seeds, and entire grains. The recommended dietary allowance (RDA) for Mg is 320 and 420 mg/d for ladies and men over age 31, individually. Intake past this sum does not appear to give further profit. A cup of spinach or Swiss chard contains around 150 mg; ¼ C of pumpkin seeds contains 190 mg; 1 C of black beans, ¾ C quinoa, and ¼ C cashews or sunflower seeds contains around 120 mg.

Oversee Stress

Stress comes in numerous structures, for example, physical (risk of threat), mental (occupation or money-related stress), and passionate (social dismissal, disconnection, or relationship stress).Stress is a characteristic and part of life and can change throughout life. On the off chance that stress gets overpowering or if there are moderate on-going stresses that are not mitigated, the body can lose its capacity to restoratively react, causing increased inflammation, which can hurt our wellbeing. The capacity to oversee stress can be created. The majority of the methodologies previously referenced eating a sound diet, being dynamic, and getting enough rest helps bolster the body's capacity to deal with life's stresses. There are extra systems that might be useful, including mind-body methodologies like care based stress reduction.

Farthest point Refined Seed Vegetable Oils

Farthest point seed oils (Soybean, corn, sunflower, safflower, grape seed, and wheat germ

Oils and processed foods, which are highly rich in omega-6 unsaturated fats, and pick sources of monounsaturated unsaturated fats, similar to olive and canola oils, while expanding the intake of omega-3-rich foods (like virus water greasy fish). The seed oils above are not intrinsically unfortunate in restricted sums. It's simply that the western diet contains a ton of them.

EXERCISE AND INFLAMMATION

It's outstanding that normal physical movement has medical advantages, including weight control, fortifying the heart, bones, and muscles and reducing the danger of specific ailments. As of late, specialists discovered how only one session of moderate exercise could likewise go about as an anti-inflammatory. The discoveries have empowering suggestions for endless illnesses like joint inflammation, fibromyalgia, and for increasingly unavoidable conditions, for example, heftiness. The examination, as of late distributed online in Brain, Behavior, and Immunity, discovered one 20-minute session of moderate exercise can invigorate the safe framework, creating an anti-inflammatory cell reaction. The cerebrum and thoughtful sensory system a pathway that serves to quicken the pulse and raise the circulatory strain, in addition to other things that are initiated during exercise to empower the body to do work. Hormones, for example, epinephrine and norepinephrine, are discharged into the circulatory system and trigger adrenergic receptors, which safe cells have. This initiation procedure during exercise produces immunological reactions, which incorporate the generation of numerous cytokines, or proteins, one of which is TNF, a key controller of nearby and foundational inflammation that likewise helps support invulnerable reactions. Studies discovered one session of around 20 minutes of moderate treadmill exercise brought about a five percent decline in the quantity of animated insusceptible cells creating TNF," "Recognizing what sets administrative components of inflammatory proteins moving may add to growing new treatments for the staggering number of people with endless inflammatory conditions, including almost 25 million Americans who experience the ill effects of immune system sicknesses. The 47 study members strolled on a treadmill at a power level that was balanced dependent on their wellness level. Blood was gathered previously and following the 20-moment exercise challenge. Exercise session doesn't really need to be serious to have anti-inflammatory effects. Twenty minutes to 30 minutes of moderate exercise, including quick strolling, gives off an impression of being adequate. Having an inclination that an exercise should be at a pinnacle effort level for a long span can threaten the individuals who experience the ill effects of constant inflammatory illnesses and could extraordinarily profit by physical action. Inflammation is an indispensable piece of the body's invulnerable reaction. It is simply the body's endeavour to recuperate after damage; guard itself against outside intruders, for example, infections and microbes; and fix harmed tissue. Nonetheless, constant inflammation can prompt genuine medical problems related to diabetes, celiac infection, corpulence, and different conditions.

The exercise starts a course of inflammatory occasions, which at last lead to long-term effects on human wellbeing. During and after intense exercise in skeletal muscle, associations between insusceptible cells, cytokines, and other intracellular components, make an inflammatory milieu in charge of the recuperation and adaption from an exercise bout. In the foundational course, cytokines discharged from muscle (myokines) intervene in metabolic and inflammatory procedures. Moderate exercise training results in upgrades in foundational irritation, apparent by decreases in intense phase proteins. The anti-inflammatory effects of normal exercise incorporate activities reliant and autonomous of changes in adipose tissue mass. Future research ought to incorporate methodologies, which endeavour to coordinate other, less-perceived physiological procedures with intense and long-term inflammatory changes. This will incorporate examination concerning metabolic, endocrine, and safe components of different tissues and organs.

SELECTED EXERCISES TO REDUCE INFLAMMATION

From running to weightlifting, physical movement is beneficial for you, to some extent, since it enables your body to battle inflammation. Presently, another survey clarifies precisely how exercise attempts to bring down inflammation. Inflammation is simply the body's method for mending after damage and shielding itself from contamination; however, incessant inflammation is connected with a wide range of illnesses, from diabetes to coronary illness. When you begin practising and moving your muscles, your muscle cells discharge a little protein called Interleukin which seems to assume a significant job in battling inflammation has a few mitigating impacts, including:

• Reducinglevels of a protein called TNF alpha, which itself actuate inflammation in the body.

- clogging the flagging impacts of a protein called interleukin 1 beta, which triggers inflammation that can harm the part in the pancreas that produces insulin. The greatest factor in deciding how much your muscles discharge is the length of your exercise, the more drawn out your exercise, the more is discharged. Here are a few exercises:

Take a walk

At the point when your body is inflamed , regardless of whether it's from exceptional exercise or something different, a light walk is a phenomenal method to reset, particularly the ones who will in general truly drive themselves, to ease up a piece and take a long walk when their body is truly fearing an intense one. Walking is an incredible method to allow your muscles to recuperate, it cuts down inflammation by sending crisp blood and oxygen all through your body, siphoning the lymphatic framework for squandering evacuation, and tenderly reestablishing your stomach related framework on the off chance that it feels off.

Foam roll

Foam roll has centre fortifying advantages; it is regularly viewed as a recuperation strategy, and for a valid justification: It assists with muscle irritation, improves adaptability, improves rest, assists with absorption, and brings down inflammation. To lessen inflammation with a foam roller, lie on a roller, and use gravity to apply strain to a muscle.

YOGA EXERCISE

This one likely doesn't come as a lot of a surprise; however, the intensity of profound breathing and yoga as an inflammation-busting strategy can't be thought little of. Profound, controlled breathing and contemplation incite a condition of physical and mental unwinding, "This is inconceivably useful when you need to bring down inflammation in the body.

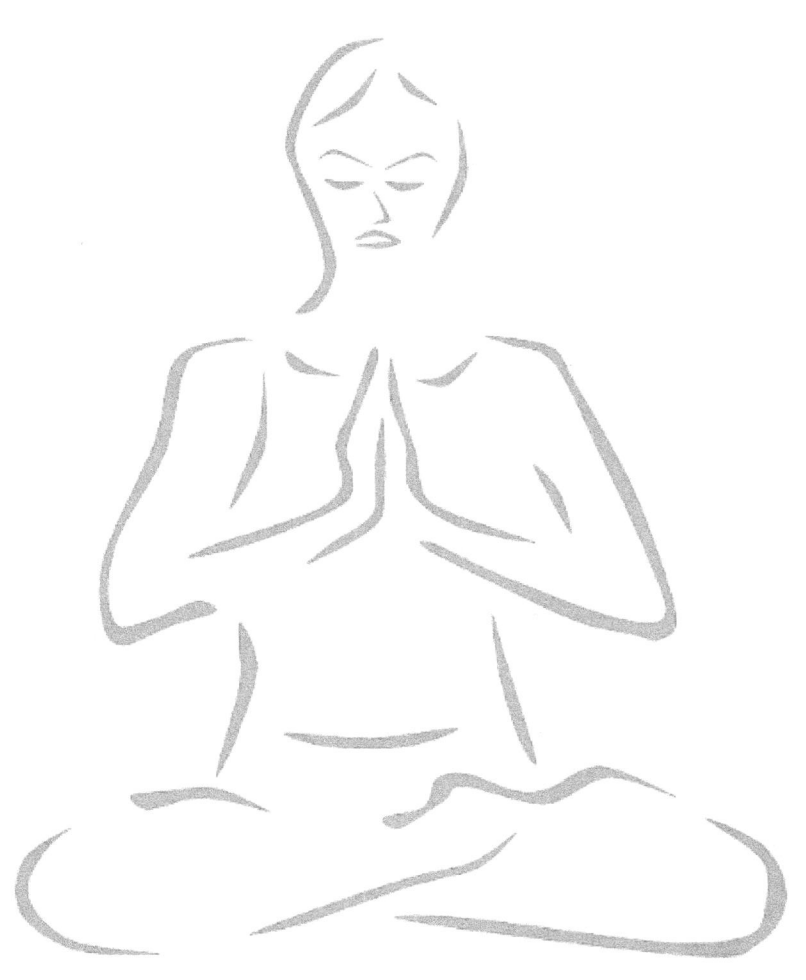

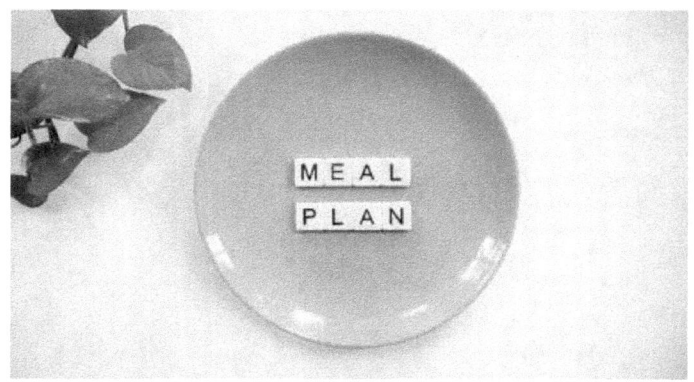

THE 21-DAY MEAL PLAN

Day 1
Breakfast - Oven-Poached Eggs
Lunch - Capellini Soup with Tofu and Shrimp
Dinner - Zucchini Endive Soup
Snacks/Desserts

Day 2
Breakfast - Breakfast Marinated Egg
Lunch - Pesto Chicken Sandwich
Dinner - Turkey Salad
Snacks/Desserts - Crostini with Tomato Spread

Day 3
Breakfast - Morning Omelette
Lunch - Chicken and Vegetable Salad with Hollandaise Sauce
Dinner - Salmon with Broccoli and Sweet Potato
Snacks/Desserts - Honey Baked Apricots

Day 4
Breakfast - Cranberry and Raisins Granola

Lunch - Iceberg Lettuce and Mushrooms Salad
Dinner - Salmon with Broccoli and Sweet Potato
Snacks/Desserts -Tapenade Crostini

Day 5
Breakfast - Cranberry and Raisins Granola
Lunch - Arugula with Gorgonzola Dressing
Dinner - Salmon with Broccoli and Sweet Potato
Snacks/Desserts - Tapenade Crostini

Day 6
Breakfast - Breakfast French Onion Soup
Lunch - Fusilli with Grape Tomatoes and Kale
Dinner - Courgettes and Peppers with Cashew Nuts
Snacks/Desserts - Baked Cinnamon Apples

Day 7
Breakfast - Spicy Marble Eggs
Lunch - Rice and Chicken Pot
Dinner - Artichoke Soup
Snacks/Desserts - Apple Chips

Day 8
Breakfast -Nutty Oats Pudding
Lunch - Shiitake and Spinach Pattie
Dinner - Mushrooms and Baby Onions
Snacks/Desserts - Blueberry Pudding

Day 9
Breakfast - Couscous with Lettuce and Carrots Salad
Lunch - Cabbage Orange Salad with Citrusy Vinaigrette
Dinner - Asparagus and Peppers Terrine
Snacks/Desserts - Chocolate Avocado Pudding

Day 10
Breakfast - Barley and Mushroom Soup
Lunch - Lemon Buttery Shrimp Rice
Dinner - Olives and Eggs Rollups
Snacks/Desserts - Banana Dark Choco Almonds

Day 11
Breakfast - Almond Pancakes with Coconut Flakes
Lunch - Valencia Salad
Dinner - Olives and Eggs Rollups
Snacks/Desserts - Honeyed Sweet Potatoes

Day 12
Breakfast - Cooled Almond Soup
Lunch - Tenderloin Stir Fry with Red and Green Grapes
Dinner - Garlic Lean Pork
Snacks/Desserts - Avocado Chia Parfait

Day 13
Breakfast - Baked Apple Turnover
Lunch - Tenderloin Stir Fry with Red and Green Grapes
Dinner - Salmon and Pickle Salad
Snacks/Desserts - Banana Cinnamon Cookies

Day 14
Breakfast - Quinoa and Cauliflower Congee
Lunch - Aioli with Eggs
Dinner - Buttered Cauliflower Mash
Snacks/Desserts - Banana Cinnamon Cookies

Day 15
Breakfast - Breakfast ArrozCaldo
Lunch - Seared Herbed Salmon Steak
Dinner - Cabbage and Fish Egg Rolls
Snacks/Desserts - Banana Cinnamon

Day 16
Breakfast - Fried Vegetable Brown Rice
Lunch - Aioli on Spaghetti Squash
Dinner - Mango Bell Pepper Salsa
Snacks/Desserts - Olive Crostini

Day 17
Breakfast - Apple Bruschetta with Almonds and Blackberries
Lunch - Vegetable Noodle Salad with Raspberry Dressing
Dinner - Chicken Barbeque Bake
Snacks/Desserts - Apple Parfait

Day 18
Breakfast - Hash Browns
Lunch - Cucumber Jicama Salad with Cashew Butter
Dinner - Crab Avocado Cilantro Salad
Snacks/Desserts - Banana Cinnamon Sandwich

Day 19
Breakfast - Romanesco Salad with Quail Eggs
Lunch - Ginger Chicken Stew
Dinner - Maple Turkey

Snacks/Desserts - Protein Crepes

Day 20
Breakfast - Romanesco Salad with Quail Eggs
Lunch - Taro Leaves in Coconut Sauce
Dinner - Artichoke Hearts Crisps
Snacks/Desserts - Sautéed Apples

Day 21
Breakfast - Asparagus and Artichoke Salad with Dijon Vinaigrette
Lunch - Buttered Prawns in Garlic Rice
Dinner - Hot Dumpling Soup
Snacks/Desserts - Apricot Cinnamon Jam

CHAPTER 1 - ANTI-INFLAMMATORY: BREAKFAST RECIPES

1. Oven-Poached Eggs

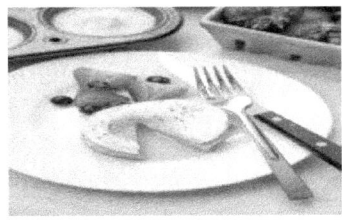

Prep Time: 2mins
Cook Time: 11mins
Total Time: 13mins
Servings: 4

Ingredients:
- 6 eggs, at room temperature
- Water
- Ice bath
- 2 cups water, chilled
- 2 cups of ice cubes

Directions:
1. Preheat oven to 175°C/350°F. Pour 2 cups of water into a deep roasting tin, and place into the lowest rack of the oven.
2. Place one egg into each cup of cupcake/muffin tins, along with one tablespoon of water.
3. Carefully place muffin tins into the middle rack of the oven.
4. Bake eggs for 45 minutes.
5. Turn off the heat immediately. Remove muffin tins from oven and set on a cake rack to cool before extracting eggs.
6. Pour ice bath ingredients into a large heat-resistant bowl.
7. Place eggs into an ice bath to stop the cooking process. After 10 minutes, drain eggs well. Use as needed.

2. Breakfast Marinated Egg

Prep Time 5 mins
Cook Time 7 mins
Inactive Prep 4 hours
Total Time 4 hours 12 mins
Servings: 4

Ingredients:
- 6, soft-cooked eggs, peeled, cooled

Marinade
- ½ cup brown sugar
- ½ cup mirin
- 1 cup of water
- 1 cup sake
- ½ cup tamari

Directions:
1. Combine marinade in a bowl. Stir until sugar dissolves.
2. Place eggs into an airtight non-reactive container just small enough to snugly fit all these in.
3. Pour in marinade. Eggs should be completely submerged in liquid. Discard leftover marinade, if any. Line container rim with generous layers of saran wrap. Secure container lid.
4. Chill eggs for 24 hours before using. Drain well after. Discard marinade.
5. Pat dry before eating, using, or storing away.

3. Breakfast Omelette

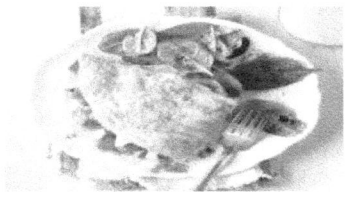

Prep: 5 mins.
Cook: 5 mins
Total Time: 10
Servings: 2

Ingredients:
- ❖ 2 eggs
- ❖ 3 egg whites
- ❖ 1 tablespoon of water
- ❖ 1/2 teaspoon of olive oil
- ❖ 1/4 teaspoon salt
- ❖ ¼ teaspoon ground pepper

Directions:
1. In a bowl, beat the eggs, egg whites, salt, pepper and water, until frothy.
2. Heat half of the oil in a skillet over medium heat. Pour half of the egg mixture. Cook for a couple of minutes, while lifting the edges using a spatula every once in a while. Fold into a half. Turn the heat to low and continue cooking for a minute.
3. Repeat the process for the rest of the egg mixture.

4. CRANBERRY AND RAISINS GRANOLA

Prep Time: 15 mins
Cook Time: 20 mins
Total Time: 35 min
Servings: 4

Ingredients:
- ❖ 4 cups old-fashioned rolled oats

- 1/4 cup sesame seeds
- 1 cup dried cranberries
- 1 cup golden raisins
- 1/8 teaspoon nutmeg
- 2 tablespoons olive oil
- 1/2 cup almonds, slivered
- 2 tablespoons warm water
- 1 teaspoon vanilla extract
- 1 teaspoon cinnamon
- 1/4 teaspoon of salt
- 6 tablespoons maple syrup
- 1/3 cup of honey

Directions:
1. In a bowl, mix the sesame seeds, nutmeg, almonds, oats, salt, and cinnamon.
2. In another bowl, mix the oil, water, vanilla, honey and syrup. Gradually pour the mixture into the oats mixture. Toss to combine. Spread the mixture into a greased jelly-roll pan. Bake in a preheated oven at 300 degrees for 55 minutes. Stir and break the clumps every 10 minutes.
3. Once you get it from the oven, stir the cranberries and raisins. Allow cooling. This will last for a week when stored in an airtight container and up to a month when stored in the fridge.

5. Breakfast French Onion Soup

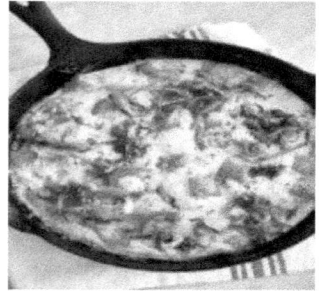

Prep time: 10 mins

Cook time: 1 hour, 10 mins
Total Time: 1 hour 20 mins
Servings: 4-6

Ingredients:
- 2 pounds onions, sliced thinly
- 1 cup chicken stock, reduced-sodium chicken broth
- 4 slices French bread, toasted
- 1 cup Swiss cheese, shredded
- 1 1/2 teaspoons Worcestershire sauce
- Freshly ground pepper
- 2 tablespoons olive oil

Directions:
1. Heat oil in a skillet over medium-high heat. Cook the onions for 15 minutes while stirring often. Remove from the stove.
2. Pour the broth in a saucepan and bring to a simmer. Add the cooked onions, pepper and Worcestershire sauce. Turn the heat to low. Simmer for 15 minutes while stirring occasionally.
3. Ladle the soup into 4 heatproof bowls. Place the bowls on a baking sheet. Put a slice of bread on top of each bowl and 1/4 cup of cheese.
4. Bake in a preheated oven at 450 degrees for 5 minutes.

6. SPICY MARBLE EGGS

Prep Time: 15 mins
Cook Time: 2 hours
Total Time: 2 hours 15 mins
Serves: 12 eggs

Ingredients:
- 6 medium-boiled eggs, unpeeled, cooled

For the Marinade
- 2 oolong black tea bags
- 3 Tbsp. brown sugar
- 1 thumb-sized fresh ginger, unpeeled, crushed
- 3 dried star anise, whole
- 2 dried bay leaves
- 3 Tbsp. light soy sauce

- ❖ 4 Tbsp. dark soy sauce
- ❖ 4 cups of water
- ❖ 1 dried cinnamon stick, whole
- ❖ 1 tsp. salt
- ❖ 1 tsp. dried Szechuan peppercorns

Directions:
1. Using the back of a metal spoon, crack eggshells in places to create a spider web effect. Do not peel. Set aside until needed.
2. Pour marinade into large Dutch oven set over high heat. Put lid partially on. Bring water to a rolling boil, about 5 minutes. Turn off heat.
3. Secure lid. Steep ingredients for 10 minutes.
4. Using a slotted spoon, fish out and discard solids. Cool marinade completely to room proceeding.
5. Place eggs into an airtight non-reactive container just small enough to snugly fit all these in.
6. Pour in marinade. Eggs should be completely submerged in liquid. Discard leftover marinade, if any. Line container rim with generous layers of saran wrap. Secure container lid.
7. Chill eggs for 24 hours before using.
8. Extract eggs and drain each piece well before using, but keep the rest submerged in the marinade.

7. *NUTTY OATS PUDDING*

Prep Time 5 mins
Total Time 5 mins
Servings 3 -5

Ingredients:
- ❖ ¼ cup rolled oats
- ❖ 1 tablespoon yoghurt, fat-free
- ❖ 1 ½ tablespoon natural peanut butter
- ❖ ¼ cup dry milk
- ❖ 1 teaspoon peanuts, finely chopped
- ❖ ½ cup of water

Directions:

1. Using a microwaveable-safe bowl, put together peanut butter and dry milk. Whisk well. Add in water to achieve a smooth consistency. Add in oats.
2. Cover bowl with plastic wrap. Create a small hole for the steam to escape.
3. Place inside the microwave oven for 1 minute on high powder.
4. Continue heating, this time on medium power for 90 seconds. Let sit for 5 minutes.
5. To serve, spoon an equal amount of cereals in a bowl top with peanuts and yoghurt.

8. Couscous with Lettuce and Carrots Salad

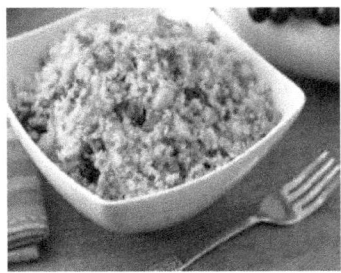

Prep Time 5 mins
Cook Tim: 15
Total Time 20 mins
Servings 3 -5

Ingredients:
- 1 cup couscous
- 2 carrots, diagonally sliced
- 2 cups baby romaine lettuce
- 1 tablespoon flaxseed oil
- ¼ teaspoon ground coriander
- 1/8 teaspoon smoked paprika
- 2 tablespoons lime juice
- 1 red bell pepper, chopped
- ¼ teaspoon ground cumin

- ❖ 4 cups of water
- ❖ 1 tablespoon extra-virgin olive oil
- ❖ Pinch of salt, add more if needed
- ❖ Pinch of pepper, add more if needed

Directions:
1. Pour 5 cups of water in a large saucepan. Bring to a boil. Add couscous. Reduce heat to low. Cover and allow simmering for 10 minutes. Stir occasionally. Drain and rinse under cold water. Set aside.
2. Meanwhile, in a mixing bowl, combine flaxseed oil, olive oil coriander, cumin, paprika, and lime juice. Whisk the mixture well.
3. Add in couscous into the mixture. Stir in red bell pepper, and carrots. Season with salt and pepper. Toss well to coat.
4. To serve, line a salad plate with lettuce. Top an equal amount of the salad.

9. BARLEY AND MUSHROOM SOUP

Prep Time: 25 mins
Cook Time: 25 mins
Total Time: 50 mins
Servings: 8

Ingredients:
- ❖ 2 onions, chopped
- ❖ 3 celery stalks, chopped
- ❖ 3 carrots, chopped
- ❖ 2 tablespoons olive oil
- ❖ 1/3 cup pearl barley
- ❖ 1/2 cup dry white wine
- ❖ Freshly ground pepper
- ❖ 9 cups reduced-sodium beef broth
- ❖ 2 to 3 tablespoons of flat-leaf parsley (minced)
- ❖ 2 10-ounce packages of mushrooms

Directions:
1. Heat oil in a saucepan over medium-high heat. Put the celery, carrots and onions. Sauté for 5 minutes. Add the wine.
2. Simmer until the cooking is reduced. Pour the broth and add the barley. Stir the mixture. Cover the saucepan and turn the heat to low. Simmer for 45 minutes while stirring occasionally.
3. Rinse the mushrooms. Cut the stems from the caps. Chop 1/3 of the caps and stems. Slice the rest of the caps.
4. Ladle 1 1/2 cups of the soup and veggies into a food processor. Process until smooth. Pour it back into the saucepan. Add the pepper, parsley and mushrooms. Stir and allow to boil. Cover the saucepan and simmer for 15 minutes.
5. Put chopped parsley on top before serving.

10. ALMOND PANCAKES WITH COCONUT FLAKES

Prep Time 5 mins
Cook Time 10 mins
Total Time 15 mins
Serves: 6

Ingredients:
- 1 overripe banana, mashed
- 2 eggs, yolks and whites separated
- ½ cup unsweetened applesauce
- 1 cup almond flour, finely milled
- ¼ cup of water
- ¼ tsp. coconut oil

Garnish
- 2 Tbsp. blanched almond flakes
- dash of cinnamon powder
- ¼ cup coconut flakes, sweetened
- pinch of sea salt
- pure maple syrup, use sparingly

Directions:
1. Whisk egg whites until soft peaks form.
2. Except for egg whites and coconut oil, combine remaining ingredients in another bowl. Mix until batter comes together.
3. Gently fold in egg whites. Make sure that you don't over mix or the pancake will become dense and chewy.
4. Pour oil into a nonstick skillet set over medium heat.

5. Wait for the oil to heat up before dropping in approximately ½ cup of batter. (Use more or less, depending on your personal preference.) Cook until edges are set, and bubbles form in the centre. Carefully flip and cook the other side for 2 more minutes.
6. Transfer flapjacks to a plate. Repeat step until all batter is cooked. Pour in more oil into the skillet only if needed. This recipe should yield between 4 to 6 medium-sized pancakes.
7. Stack pancakes. Pour the desired amount of pure maple syrup on top. Garnish each stack with cinnamon-flavoured almond-coconut flakes just before serving.
8. For the garnish, preheat oven to 350°F (175°C) for at least 10 minutes prior to use. Line a baking sheet with parchment paper. Set aside.
9. Mix almond and coconut flakes together in a bowl. Spread mixture evenly on a prepared baking sheet.
10. Bake for 7 to 10 minutes until flakes turn golden brown. Stir almond and coconut flakes once midway through roasting to prevent over-browning.

Remove baking sheet from oven. Cool almond and coconut flakes for at least 10 minutes before sprinkling in cinnamon powder and salt. Toss to combine. Set aside.

11. COOLED ALMOND SOUP

Prep time: 5 mins
Cook time: 5 mins
Total time: 10 mins
Servings: 4

Ingredients:
- 2 garlic cloves, sliced
- 4 slices bread, crust removed
- 5 teaspoons apple cider vinegar
- 1 cup blanched almonds
- 3 cups chilled water
- 5 tablespoons olive oil

For garnish
- Toasted flaked almonds
- Grapes, seedless

Directions:
1. Break bread in a bowl. Pour over chilled water. Leave for 5 minutes.

2. Combine almonds and garlic in a blender. Process until finely ground. Add the soaked bread. Process until smooth.
3. Gradually put the oil until the mixture forms a smooth paste. Add sherry vinegar and the remaining chilled water. Process until smooth
4. Season with salt and pepper. Chill in the fridge for 3 hours.
5. Ladle the soup into a chilled bowl. Scatter with almonds and grapes. Serve.

12. BAKED APPLE TURNOVER

Prep Time: 30 mins
Cook Time: 25 mins
Total Time: 55 mins
Servings: 4

Ingredients:

For the turnovers
- 4 apples, peeled, cored, diced into bite-sized pieces
- 1 Tbsp. almond flour
- all-purpose flour, for rolling out the dough
- 1 frozen puff pastry, thawed
- ½ cup palm sugar, crumbled by hand to loosen granules
- ½ tsp. cinnamon powder

For the egg wash
- 1 egg white, whisked in
- 2 Tbsp. water

Directions:
1. For the filling: combine almond flour, cinnamon powder and palm sugar until these resemble coarse meal. Toss in diced apples until well coated. Set aside.
2. On a lightly floured surface, roll out the puff pastry until ¼ inch thin. Slice into 8 pieces of 4" x 4" squares.
3. Divide prepared apples into 8 equal portions. Spoon on individual puff pastry squares. Fold in half diagonally. Press edges to seal.
4. Place each filled pastry on a baking tray lined with parchment paper. Make sure there is ample space in between pastries.
5. Freeze for at least 20 minutes, or until ready to bake.
6. Preheat oven to 400°F or 205°C for at 10 minutes.
7. Brush frozen pastries with egg wash. Place in a hot oven, and cook for 12 to 15 minutes, or until these turn golden brown all over.

8. Remove baking tray from oven immediately. Cool slightly for easier handling.
9. Place 1 apple turnover on a plate. Serve warm.

13. QUINOA AND CAULIFLOWER CONGEE

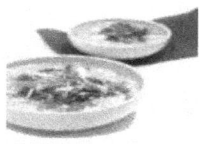

Prep Time: 10 mins
Cook Time: 1 hr
Total Time: 1 hr 10 mins
Serves: 8

Ingredients:

- 1 cauliflower head, minced
- 2 tablespoons red quinoa
- 2 leeks, minced
- 1 tablespoon fresh ginger, grated
- 2 garlic cloves, grated
- 6 cups of water
- 2 tablespoons brown rice
- 1 tablespoon olive oil
- 1 tablespoon fish sauce
- 2 onions, minced
- Pinch of white pepper

For Garnish

- 4 eggs, soft-boiled
- 2 red chili, minced
- 1 lime, sliced into wedges
- ¼ cup packed basil leaves, torn

- ❖ ¼ cup loosely packed cilantro leaves, torn
- ❖ ¼ cup loosely packed spearmint leaves, torn

Directions:
1. Pour olive oil into a large skillet set over medium heat. Sauté shallots, garlic, and ginger until limp and aromatic; pour into a slow cooker set at medium heat.
2. Except for garnishes, pour remaining ingredients into slow cooker; stir. Put the lid on. Cook for 6 hours. Turn off heat. Taste; adjust seasoning if needed.
3. Ladle congee into individual bowls. Garnish with basil leaves, cilantro leaves, red chili, and spearmint leaves. Add 1 piece of soft-boiled egg on top of each; serve with a wedge of lime on the side. Slice egg just before eating so yolk runs into congee. Squeeze lime juice into congee just before eating.

14. BREAKFAST ARROZCALDO

Prep Time: 20 mins
Cook Time: 30 mins
Total Time: 50 mins
Servings: 5

Ingredients:

- ❖ 6 eggs, white only
- ❖ 1½ cups brown rice, cooked

For the filling

- ❖ ¼ cup raisins
- ❖ ½ cup frozen peas, thawed
- ❖ 1 white onion, minced
- ❖ 1 garlic clove, minced
- ❖ oil, for greasing

Directions:
1. For the filling, spray a small amount of oil into a skillet set over medium heat. Add in onion and garlic. Stir-fry until former is limp and transparent.

2. Stir-fry while breaking up clumps, about 2 minutes. Add in remaining ingredients. Stir-fry for another minute.
3. Turn down the heat, and let filling cook for 10 to 15 minutes, or until juices are greatly reduced. Stir often. Turn off heat. Divide into 6 equal portions.
4. For the eggs, spray a small amount of oil into a smaller skillet set over medium heat. Cook eggs. Discard yolk. Transfer to holding the plate.
5. To serve, place 1 portion of rice on a plate, along with 1 portion of filling, and 1 egg white. Serve warm.

15. FRIED VEGETABLE BROWN RICE

Prep Time 5 mins
Cook Time 10 mins
Total Time 15 mins

Ingredients:

- ❖ 4 cups brown rice, cooked
- ❖ 1 ½ cups carrots, diced
- ❖ ¾ cup celery, diced
- ❖ 1 ½ cup green onions, chopped
- ❖ 1 ½ Tbsp. garlic, minced
- ❖ ¾ cup red bell pepper, diced
- ❖ 3 Tbsp. fresh chilies, minced
- ❖ 3 Tbsp. fresh cilantro, chopped
- ❖ 1 red bell pepper, diced
- ❖ 1 ½ Tbsp. soy sauce
- ❖ 3 tsp. sesame oil
- ❖ Ground white pepper, to taste
- ❖ 3 Tbsp. olive oil

Directions:
1. Place the wok over high flame and heat through. Add the vegetable oil and swirl to coat.
2. Stir in the shallots, garlic, and chilies until fragrant, then add the carrots and reduce to medium flame. Sauté until crisp-tender.
3. Stir in the rice, celery, and bell pepper and mix well. Pour in the soy sauce and season with the salt and white pepper.

4. Stir fry until the rice is broken down and heated through. Fold in the cilantro and transfer to a serving dish. Drizzle with sesame oil and serve right away.

16. APPLE BRUSCHETTA WITH ALMONDS AND BLACKBERRIES

Ingredients:
- 1 apple, sliced into ¼-inch thick half-moons
- ¼ cup blackberries, thawed, lightly mashed
- ½ tsp. fresh lemon juice
- ⅛ cup almond slivers, toasted
- sea salt

Directions:
1. Drizzle lemon juice on apple slices. Place these on a tray lined with parchment paper.
2. Spread a small number of mashed berries on top of each slice. Top these off with the desired amount of almond slivers.
3. Sprinkle sea salt on "bruschetta" just before serving.

17. HASH BROWNS

Prep Time: 15 mins
Cook Time: 15 mins
Total Time: 30 mins
Servings: 4

Ingredients:
- 1 pound Russet potatoes, peeled, processed using a grater
- Pinch of sea salt
- Pinch of black pepper, to taste
- 3 Tbsp. olive oil

Directions:
1. Line a microwave safe-dish with paper towels. Spread shredded potatoes on top. Microwave veggies on highest heat setting for 2 minutes. Remove from heat.
2. Pour 1 tablespoon of oil into a non-stick skillet set over medium heat.
3. Cooking in batches, place a generous pinch of potatoes into the hot oil. Press down using the back of a spatula.
4. Cook for 3 minutes on each side, or until brown and crispy. Drain on paper towels. Repeat step for remaining potatoes. Add more oil as needed.
5. Season with salt and pepper. Serve.

18. Cucumber Jicama Salad with Cashew Butter

Prep Time: 10 mins
Total Time; 10 mins:
Servings: 4

Ingredients

For Salad
- 1 jicama, sliced into ¼-inch thick matchsticks
- 1 celery stalk, julienned
- 2 cucumbers, sliced into ¼-inch thick matchsticks
- Pinch of sea salt
- Pinch of black pepper, to taste
- 4 Tbsp. cashew butter

For cashew butter
- 1 cup cashew nuts, toasted, cooled before processing
- Pinch of sea salt
- 1 Tbsp. coconut oil, melted

Directions:
For salad
1. Toss ingredients into the salad bowl to combine.
2. Chill for 15 minutes before serving.

For cashew butter
1. Place ingredients of cashew butter into a blender. Process until smooth, scraping down sides of blender often.

19. ROMANESCO SALAD WITH QUAIL EGGS

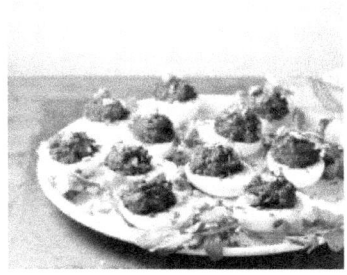

Prep Time: 15 mins
Cook Time: 5mins
Servings: 6

Ingredients:
- 1 avocado, mashed
- 12 pieces quail eggs, hard-boiled, halved
- 2 green Romanesco salad tomatoes, chopped
- 1 raw egg yolk
- 2 red Romanesco salad tomatoes, chopped
- 1 lemon, freshly squeezed
- Pinch of sea salt
- Pinch of white pepper, to taste

Directions:
1. Combine avocado, egg yolk, and lemon juice in a bowl; season well with salt and pepper.
2. Place remaining ingredients into a salad bowl. Drizzle in the avocado-lemon mix.
3. Toss salad to combine. Serve.

20. ASPARAGUS AND ARTICHOKE SALAD WITH DIJON VINAIGRETTE

Prep Time : 10 mins
Cook Time: 2 hrs

Total Time: 2 hrs 10 mins
Servings: 6

Ingredients:
- 1 cup asparagus spears, cooked
- 1 cup artichoke hearts, cooked
- 1 egg, hard-boiled, chopped finely
- 1 tablespoon thyme, chopped
- 2 garlic cloves, minced
- 2 tablespoons chicken stock, reduced-sodium
- 1 tablespoon cider vinegar
- 1 tablespoon Dijon mustard
- 1 teaspoon of dry mustard
- 1 tablespoon of flat-leaf parsley, minced
- 1/4 teaspoon of salt
- Freshly ground pepper
- 4 teaspoons of olive oil

Directions:
1. Arrange the cooked asparagus, artichoke hearts and green beans on a platter.
2. Put the vinegar, broth, dry mustard, Dijon mustard, pepper, thyme, salt and garlic, in a blender or food processor. Stire the mixture over the veggies.
3. Put parsley and egg on top of your salad. Cover with plastic wrap and put in the fridge for at least 8 hours. Leave at room temperature for half an hour before serving.

21. BARLEY APPLE SALAD

Prep Time 10 mins
Cook Time 15 mins
Total Time 7 hours 25 mins
Servings 4

Ingredients:

- 2/3 cup pearl barley
- 1 slightly tart apple, cored, cubed
- 3 tablespoons sweet onion, diced
- 1 tablespoon fresh orange juice
- 1 cup of green seedless grapes, halved
- 2 tablespoons mayonnaise
- 3 cups of water
- 1/2 teaspoon of sugar
- 1 tablespoon fresh lemon juice
- 3/4 teaspoon of salt
- 1/4 cup of plain yoghurt
- 1/3 cup of pecan, halved, chopped

Directions:
1. Put water, salt and barley in a saucepan over medium-high heat. Bring to a boil. Turn the heat to low and cover the saucepan. Simmer for 30 minutes. Drain. Rinse the barley in cold water.
2. In a bowl, mix the mayonnaise, sugar, tangerine juice, lemon juice and yoghurt. Add the grapes, apple and barley. Toss to coat.
3. You can sprinkle the salad with pecans before serving.

22. CUCUMBER AND PEPPER SALAD

Prep Time: 10mins
Cook Time: 3hrs
Total Time: 3hrs10
Servings: 8

Ingredients:

- 1 cucumber, julienned
- 1 red bell pepper, julienned
- 1 leek, white part only, julienned
- 1 jicama, julienned
- 1 Thai chili, deseeded, julienned

Dressing

- 1 tsp. balsamic vinegar
- ¼ cup apple cider vinegar

- 1 garlic, grated
- 1 bird's eye chili, minced
- 1 tsp. fresh cilantro, minced
- 1/8 cup extra virgin olive oil
- Pinch of sea salt
- Pinch of black pepper to taste
- Dash of red pepper flakes

Directions:
1. Pour dressing ingredients into a bottle with a tight-fitting lid. Shake until dressing emulsifies.
2. Toss salad ingredients into a bowl; drizzle in half of the dressing. Toss to combine. Place a generous portion of salad on a plate. Add more dressing only if needed. Serve.

23. POTATOES AND LEEKS SOUP

Prep time: 20 mins
Cook time: 40 mins
Total Time: 1 hr
Servings: 4-6

Ingredients:
- 6 potatoes, peeled, chopped
- 3 leeks, sliced thinly
- 2 cups chicken stock
- Pinch of ground pepper

Directions:
1. Pour the broth in a saucepan over medium-high heat. Add the leeks, pepper and potatoes.
2. Cover the saucepan and simmer for 30 minutes. Turn off the heat. Allow cooling slightly.
3. Put all or 2 cups of the veggies, depending on your preferred texture, in a food processor.
4. Add 2 cups of broth. Process until smooth. Put the mixture back to the saucepan and stir. Reheat.

24. Sun-Dried Tomato Garlic Bruschetta

Prep Time: 10minutes
Cook Time: 5minutes
Servings: 6

Ingredients
- 2 slices sourdough bread, toasted
- 1 tsp. chives, minced
- 1 garlic clove, peeled
- 2 tsp. sun-dried tomatoes in olive oil, minced
- 1 tsp. olive oil

Directions:
1. Vigorously rub garlic clove on 1 side of each of the toasted bread slices
2. Spread equal portions of sun-dried tomatoes on garlic side of bread. Sprinkle chives and drizzle olive oil on top.
3. Pop both slices into oven toaster, and cook until well heated through.
4. Place bruschetta on a plate. Serve warm.

25. Mushroom Crêpes

Prep Time: 1 hour 30 minutes
Cook Time: 30 minutes
Total Time: 2 hours
Servings: 6

Ingredients:
- 2 eggs
- 3/4 cup milk
- 1/2 cup all-purpose flour
- 1/4 teaspoon salt

For the filling
- 3 tablespoons all-purpose flour
- 2 cups of cremini mushrooms, sliced
- 3/4 cup chicken broth
- 1/2 cup Parmesan cheese, grated

- ❖ 1/8 teaspoon cayenne
- ❖ 1/8 teaspoon nutmeg
- ❖ ¾ cup milk
- ❖ 3 garlic cloves, minced
- ❖ 2 tablespoons of parsley (chopped)
- ❖ 6 slices of deli-sliced cooked lean ham
- ❖ 1/4 teaspoon of salt
- ❖ Freshly ground pepper

Directions:
1. Combine the salt and flour in a bowl. In another bowl, whisk the eggs and milk. Gradually combine the two mixtures until smooth. Leave for 15 minutes.
2. Spray a skillet with non-stick cooking spray and put over medium heat. Stir the batter a little. Pour 1/4 of the batter into the skillet. Tilt the skillet to form a thin and even crêpe. Cook for a couple of minutes or until the bottom is golden and the top is set. Flip and cook for 20 seconds. Transfer to a plate.
3. Repeat the steps with the remaining batter. Loosely cover the cooked crêpes with plastic wrap.
4. For the filling. Put the following in a saucepan over medium heat – flour, milk, cayenne, nutmeg, and pepper. Constantly whisk until thick or around 7 minutes. Remove from the stove. Stir in a tablespoon of parsley and cheese. Loosely cover to keep warm.
5. Spray a skillet with non-stick cooking spray and put over medium heat. Cook the garlic and mushrooms. Season with salt. Cook for 6 minutes or until the mushrooms are soft. Add 2 tablespoons of sherry. Cook for a couple of minutes. Remove from the stove. Add the remaining parsley and stir.
6. Put the crêpes side by side on a flat surface. Spread a tablespoon of the sauce and 2 tablespoons of the cooked mushrooms. Roll up the crêpes and transfer them to a greased baking dish. Pour the rest of the sauce on top. Bake in a preheated oven at 450 degrees for 15 minutes.

Chapter 2 - Anti-Inflammatory: Lunch Recipes

26. Capellini Soup with Tofu and Shrimp

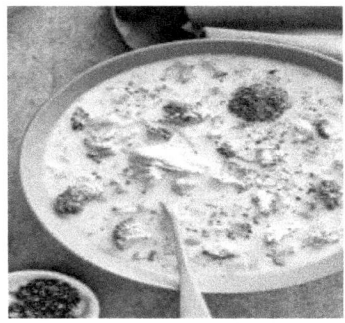

Prep Time: 20 mins
Cook Time: 20 mins
Total Time: 40 min
Servings: 8

Ingredients:
- 4 cups of bok choy, sliced
- 1/4 pound shrimp, peeled, deveined
- 1 block firm tofu, sliced into squares
- 1 can sliced water chestnuts, drained
- 1 bunch scallions, sliced
- 2 cups reduced-sodium chicken broth
- 2 teaspoons soy sauce, reduced-sodium
- 2 cups capellini
- 2 teaspoons of sesame oil
- Freshly ground white pepper
- 1 teaspoon of rice wine vinegar

Directions:
1. 1. Pour the broth in a saucepan over medium-high heat. Bring to a boil. Add the shrimp, bok choy, oil and sauce. Allow to boil and turn the heat to low. Simmer for 5 minutes.
2. 2. Add the water chestnuts, pepper, vinegar, tofu, capellini and scallions. Cook for 5 minutes or until the capellini is barely tender. Serve while hot.

27. Chicken and Vegetable Salad with Hollandaise Sauce

Prep Time: 20 mins
Cook Time: 30 mins
Total Time: 50 mins
Servings: 6

Ingredients:

For salad
- 2 large tomatoes, deseeded, diced
- ½ cup red chard leaves, choose small leaves only, rinsed, spun-dried
- 2 cups boiled/roasted chicken, diced, leftovers are fine
- 2 cups green Romaine lettuce, roughly torn, rinsed, spun-dried
- 1 small celery, skin scrubbed clean, deseeded, diced

For hollandaise sauce
- 2 pieces, large egg yolks at room temperature
- ⅛ tsp. Spanish paprika powder
- 3 Tbsp. coconut oil, heated
- 1 Tbsp. lemon juice, freshly squeezed at room temperature
- ½ tsp. kosher salt

Directions:
1. For the sauce, process egg yolks and lemon juice in the blender until smooth. With the machine running, pour warmed coconut oil in a slow, steady stream.
2. Add in remaining ingredients and process until smooth.
3. Place salad ingredients into a large bowl. Drizzle in half of the hollandaise sauce. Toss well to combine.
4. Spoon equal portions of salad into plates; drizzle equal portion of remaining dressings on top. Serve.

28. Iceberg Lettuce and Mushrooms Salad

Prep Time: 10 mins
Cook Time: 20 mins
Total Time: 30 mins
Servings : 4

Ingredients:
- 1 head, large iceberg lettuce, sliced into 6 equal wedges, retain a core, rinsed, spun-dried

For the dressing
- 1 can, 15 oz. button mushroom, stems and pieces, rinsed, drained well
- 1 cup Greek yoghurt
- ¼ cup cottage cheese
- 2 Tbsp. lemon juice, freshly squeezed
- ½ cup white wine vinegar
- ½ tsp. black pepper
- ¼ tsp. green stevia

Directions:
1. Except for button mushrooms, combine all dressing ingredients in a bowl. Mix until creamy. If dressing is too thick, add more vinegar. Fold in mushrooms. Divide into 6 equal portions.
2. Place 1 wedge of lettuce wedge on a plate. Top with 1 portion of the dressing

29. Arugula with Gorgonzola Dressing

Total Time: 10 mins
Prep Time: 10 mins
Servings: 4

Ingredients:
- 1 bunch of arugula, cleaned
- 1 pear, sliced thinly
- 1 tablespoon fresh lemon juice
- 1 garlic clove, bruised
- 1/3 cup Gorgonzola cheese, crumbled

- 1/4 cup vegetable stock, reduced-sodium
- Freshly ground pepper
- 4 teaspoons olive oil
- 1 tablespoon of cider vinegar

Directions:
1. 1. Put the pear slices and lemon juice in a bowl. Toss to coat. Arrange the slices, along with the arugula, on a platter.
2. 2. In a bowl, combine the vinegar, oil, cheese, broth, pepper and garlic. Leave for 5 minutes. Remove the garlic. Drizzle the dressing on top of the salad, and serve.

30. FUSILLI WITH GRAPE TOMATOES AND KALE

Prep Time: 15 Mins
Cook Time: 15 mins
Total Time: 30 Mins
Serves : 4

Ingredients:
- ¼ cup wholegrain fusilli, cooked according to package instructions
- 1 handful kale, sliced into bite-sized pieces
- ½ cup grape tomatoes, quartered
- 2 Tbsp. cooking liquid
- ½ Tbsp. olive oil
- ¼ cup leeks, thinly sliced
- 1 garlic clove, minced
- Pinch of sea salt
- Pinch of black pepper, to taste
- 1 tsp., roasted almonds, chopped
- pecorino cheese, grated, for sprinkling

Directions:
1. Pour oil into a saucepan set over high heat. Add in leeks and garlic. Turn down the heat and sauté until leeks are soft, about 2 minutes.
2. Add in kale and tomatoes. Stir often until kale is wilted, about 4 minutes.
3. Except for cheese, add in remaining ingredients. Toss well to combine.
4. Place pasta dish on a plate and sprinkle pecorino cheese on top. Serve.

31. Rice and Chicken Pot

Prep Time: 5 mins
Cook Time: 25 mins
Total Time: 30 mins
Servings: 4

Ingredients:
- 1 lb free-range chicken breast, boneless, skinless
- ¼ cup of brown rice
- ¾ lb mushrooms of choice, sliced
- 1 leek, chopped
- ¼ cup almonds, chopped
- 1 cup of water
- 1 Tbsp. olive oil
- 1 cup green beans
- ½ cup apple cider vinegar
- 2 Tbsp. all-purpose flour
- 1 cup milk, low fat
- ¼ cup Parmesan cheese, freshly grated
- ¼ cup sour cream
- Pinch of sea salt, add more if needed
- ground black pepper, to taste

Directions:
1. Pour brown rice into a pot. Add in water. Cover and bring to a boil. Reduce heat and allow to simmer for 30 minutes or until rice is cooked.
2. Meanwhile, in a skillet, add the chicken breast and pour just enough water to cover. Season with salt. Bring mixture to a boil then reduce heat and allow to simmer for 10 minutes or until cooked through.
3. Shred the chicken. Set aside.
4. In the same skillet, heat the olive oil. Cook leeks until tender. Add in mushrooms.
5. Pour apple cider vinegar into the mixture. Sauté the mixture until the vinegar has evaporated. Add in flour and milk into the skillet. Sprinkle Parmesan cheese and add in sour cream. Season with black pepper.
6. Preheat the oven at 350 degrees F. lightly grease a casserole dish with oil.

7. Spread cooked rice in the casserole dish. Spread shredded chicken and green beans on top. Add mushrooms and leeks sauce. Put almonds on top.
8. Bake for 20 minutes or until golden brown. Allow cooling before serving.

32. SHIITAKE AND SPINACH PATTIE

Prep Time: 10 mins
Cook Time: 15 mins
Total Time: 25 mins
Servings: 8

Ingredients:
- 1 ½ cups shiitake mushrooms, minced
- 1 ½ cups spinach, chopped
- 3 garlic cloves, minced
- 2 onions, minced
- 4 tsp. olive oil
- 1 egg
- 1 ½ cups quinoa, cooked
- 1 ½ tsp. Italian seasoning
- 1/3 cup toasted sunflower seeds, ground
- 1/3 cup Pecorino cheese, grated

Directions:
1. Heat olive oil in a saucepan. Once hot, saute shiitake mushrooms for 3 minutes or until lightly seared. Add in garlic and onion. Saute for 2 minutes or until fragrant and translucent. Set aside.
2. In the same saucepan, heat the remaining olive oil. Add in spinach. Reduce heat. Allow to simmer for 1 minute, or until the spinach is wilted. Drain and transfer to a strainer.
3. Chop spinach finely and add into the mushroom mixture. Add egg into the spinach mixture. Fold in cooked quinoa. Season with Italian seasoning. Mix until well combined. Sprinkle sunflower seeds and cheese.
4. Divide the spinach mixture into patties. Cook patties in the skillet for 5 minutes or until firm and golden brown. Serve with burger bread.

33. Cabbage Orange Salad with Citrusy Vinaigrette

Prep Time: 10 mins
Cook Time: 0 mins
Total Time: 10 mins
Servings: 8

Ingredients:
- 1 teaspoon orange zest, grated
- 2 tablespoons vegetable stock, reduced-sodium
- 1 teaspoon each cider vinegar
- 4 cups red cabbage, shredded
- 1 teaspoon lemon juice
- 1 fennel bulb, sliced thinly
- 1 teaspoon balsamic vinegar
- 1 teaspoon raspberry vinegar
- 2 tablespoons of fresh orange juice
- 2 oranges, peeled, sliced into pieces
- 1 tablespoon of honey
- 1/4 teaspoon of salt
- Freshly ground pepper
- 4 teaspoons of olive oil

Directions:
1. Put the following in a bowl and whisk – lemon juice, orange zest, cider vinegar, salt and pepper, broth, oil, honey, orange juice, balsamic vinegar and raspberry vinegar.
2. Extract the oranges, fennel and cabbage. Toss to coat.

34. Lemon Buttery Shrimp Rice

Ingredients:
- ¼ cup wild rice, cooked according to package instructions
- ½ tsp. butter, divided
- ¼ tsp. olive oil
- 1 cup raw shrimps, shelled, deveined, drained
- ¼ cup frozen peas, thawed, rinsed, drained
- 1 Tbsp. lemon juice, freshly squeezed
- 1 Tbsp. chives, minced

- ❖ Pinch of sea salt, to taste

Directions:
1. Pour ¼ tsp. butter and oil into wok set over medium heat. Add in shrimps and peas. Sauté until shrimps are coral pink, about 5 to 7 minutes.
2. Add in wild rice and cook until well heated through. Season with salt and butter.
3. Transfer to a plate. Sprinkle chives and lemon juice on top. Serve.

35. *VALENCIA SALAD*

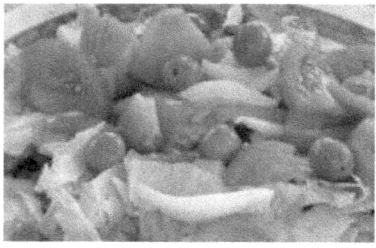

Prep Time: 10 mins
Cook Time: 0 mins
Total Time: 10
Servings: 10

Ingredients:
- ❖ 1 tsp. Kalamata olives in oil, pitted, drained lightly, halved, julienned
- ❖ 1 head, small Romaine lettuce, rinsed, spun-dried, sliced into bite-sized pieces
- ❖ ½ piece, small shallot, julienned
- ❖ 1 tsp. Dijon mustard
- ❖ ½ small satsuma or tangerine, pulp only
- ❖ 1 tsp. white wine vinegar
- ❖ 1 tsp. extra virgin olive oil
- ❖ 1 pinch fresh thyme, minced
- ❖ Pinch of sea salt
- ❖ Pinch of black pepper, to taste

Directions:
1. Combine vinegar, oil, fresh thyme, salt, mustard, black pepper, and honey, if using. Whisk well until dressing emulsifies a little.
2. Toss together remaining salad ingredients in a salad bowl.
3. Drizzle dressing on top when about to serve. Serve immediately with 1 slice if sugar-free sourdough bread or saltine.

36. TENDERLOIN STIR FRY WITH RED AND GREEN GRAPES

Prep Time: 15 mins
Cook Time: 25 mins
Total Time: 40 mins
Servings: 4

Ingredients:
- 1 medallion, 6 oz. pork tenderloin, trimmed well, remove membrane
- sea salt
- sesame oil

For grape vinaigrette
- ¼ cup green grapes, quartered
- ¼ cup red grapes, quartered
- black peppercorns, freshly cracked
- 1 tsp. apple cider vinegar, freshly juiced

Directions:
1. To make the vinaigrette, toss ingredients in a bowl. Chill prior to serving.
2. Meanwhile, preheat stovetop or electric grill for at least 3 minutes.
3. Lightly season pork with salt and sesame oil. Grill only until well seared on both sides, about 10 to 12 minutes. Remove from grill. Tent with aluminium foil, and allow the meat to rest 5 minutes.
4. Place cooked pork medallion on a plate. Top off with vinaigrette. Serve.

37. AIOLI WITH EGGS

Prep Time: 20 mins
Total Time: 20 mins
Servings: 12

Ingredients:
- 2 egg yolks
- 1 garlic, grated
- 2 Tbsp. water
- ½ cup extra virgin olive oil
- ¼ cup lemon juice, fresh squeezed, pips removed
- ¼ tsp. sea salt
- Dash of cayenne pepper powder
- Pinch of white pepper, to taste

Directions:
1. Pour garlic, egg yolks, salt and water into blender; process until smooth. Drizzle in olive oil in a slow stream until dressing emulsifies.
2. Add in remaining ingredients. Taste; adjust seasoning if needed. Pour into an airtight container; use as needed.

38. AIOLI ON SPAGHETTI SQUASH

Prep Time:10 mins
Cook Time: 10 mins
Total Time: 20 mins
Serving: 4

Ingredients:
- 1 spaghetti squash, halved lengthwise, seeds scooped out
- ¼ cup Aioli with eggs
- olive oil for drizzling
- sea salt
- black pepper to taste

Directions:
1. Preheat oven to 375°F/190°C. Line rimmed baking sheet with parchment paper. Using a pastry brush, lightly grease baking sheet with oil.
2. Drizzle more oil onto cut sides of squash, with a generous sprinkling of salt and pepper.

3. Place veggies cut side down on baking sheet; roast in a hot oven for 40 to 45 minutes or until squash is fork-tender.
4. Remove from heat; cool completely to room temperature. Flip squash over; fork through flesh to make spaghetti strands.
5. Place veggie noodles in a bowl; pour in ¼ cup of aioli. Toss gently to combine. Taste; drizzle in more aioli if desired. Season well salt and pepper if desired; serve.

39. VEGETABLE NOODLE SALAD WITH RASPBERRY DRESSING

Prep Time: 35mins
Cook Time: 10 mins
Total Time: 45 mins
Servings: 4

Ingredients:
- 1 cup raspberries, halved, for garnish

Salad
- 1 cucumber, ends trimmed, processed into flat noodles using *spiralizer* or vegetable peeler
- 2 heads oak leaf lettuce, sliced into 2-inch long slivers, rinsed, spun-dried
- 1 zucchini, ends trimmed, processed into flat noodles using *spiralizer* or vegetable peeler
- 1 head arugula, sliced into 2-inch long slivers, rinsed, spun-dried

Dressing
- 4 frozen raspberries, thawed, minced
- 1 jalapeño pepper, minced
- 1 Thai green chili, deseeded, minced
- 1 tsp. Dijon or yellow mustard
- ½ cup extra virgin olive oil
- ⅛ cup apple cider vinegar
- ⅛ cup raspberry vinegar
- Pinch of sea salt
- Pinch of black pepper to taste

Directions:
1. Place dressing ingredients into a bottle with a tight-fitting lid; shake until dressing emulsifies.
2. Place salad ingredients in a bowl; season with half of the vinaigrette. Toss to combine.

3. Spoon salad into plates and top each off with equal amounts of raspberries. Season with more dressing if desired; serve.

40. Ginger Chicken Stew

Prep Time: 10mins
Cook Time: 20mins
Total Time: 30mins
Servings: 4-6

Ingredients:
- ¼ cup chicken thigh fillet, diced
- ¼ cup cooked egg noodles
- 1 unripe papaya, peeled, diced
- 1 cup chicken broth, low-sodium, low-fat
- 1 medallion ginger, peeled, crushed
- dash onion powder
- dash garlic powder, add more if desired
- 1 cup of water
- 1 tsp. fish sauce
- dash white pepper
- 1 piece, small bird's eye chili, minced

Directions:
1. Place all ingredients in a large Dutch oven set over high heat. Let the liquid come to a full boil. Turn down heat to the lowest setting. Put the lid on.
2. Let the stew cook for 20 minutes, or until papaya is fork-tender. Turn off heat. Consume as is, or with ½ cup of cooked rice. Serve warm.

41. Taro Leaves in Coconut Sauce

Prep Time: 10 mins
Cook Time: 20 mins
Total Time: 35 mins
Servings: 5

Ingredients:
- 4 cups dried taro leaves
- 2 cans of coconut cream, divided

- ❖ ¼ cup ground pork, 90% lean
- ❖ 1 tsp. shrimp paste
- ❖ 1 bird's eye chili, minced

Directions:
1. Except for 1 can of coconut cream, place all ingredients in a crockpot set at medium setting. Secure lid. Cook undisturbed for 3 to 3½ hours.
2. Pour remaining can of coconut cream before turning off the heat. Stir and serve.

42. BUTTERED PRAWNS IN GARLIC RICE

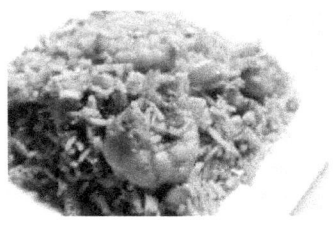

Prep Time : 10 mins
Cook Time : 15 mins
Total Time: 25
Serves : 2

Ingredients:
- ❖ ½ cup cooked brown or wild
- ❖ 4 tiger prawns, shelled, deveined, halved lengthwise
- ❖ 1 garlic, minced
- ❖ ⅛ tsp. butter
- ❖ ⅛ tsp. olive oil
- ❖ sea salt

Directions:
1. Pour oil in a wok set over high heat. Sauté butter until golden and aromatic. Do not burn. Remove from wok immediately.
2. In the same wok, stir-fry prawns until these turn coral, about 3 minutes. Season well.
3. Add in remaining ingredients, including garlic. Cook until rice is heated through, about 3 more minutes. Serve warm.

43. Pesto Chicken Sandwich

Prep Time: 15 mins
Cook Time: 1hr 30mins
Serving: 4

Ingredients:

For the Pesto
- 3 garlic cloves, chopped
- 1 cup fresh basil leaves
- 2 Tbsp. pine nuts, freshly toasted
- Pinch of sea salt, add more if needed
- Pinch of black pepper, to taste
- $1/3$ cup extra virgin olive oil
- $1/3$ cup cashew cheese
- 4 pieces of bread, halved
- olive oil, for brushing

For the Toppings
- 2 cups chicken breast, cooked, shredded
- 2 cups arugula leaves
- 1 beefsteak tomato, sliced into thick medallions
- ¼ cup cashew cheese

Directions:
1. For the bread, lightly coat sides of the bread with olive oil. Toast in an oven toaster. Set aside.
2. For the pesto, put garlic cloves, basil leaves, pine nuts, salt, and black pepper into a blender. Process several times until basil leaves are minced.
3. Pour olive oil and cashew cheese into the blender. Process until the desired consistency is achieved. Adjust taste if needed.
4. To serve, put together shredded chicken and an equal amount of pesto in a bowl. Mix well.
5. Spread cashew cheese on toasted wheat bread. Layer with arugula leaves, chicken, and tomato slices. Top off with the other bread slice. Serve.

44. Pepper Stuffed Quinoa

Prep Time: 10 mins
Cook Time: 1 hour 5 mins
Total Time: 1 hour 15 mins
Servings: 4

Ingredients:

For the Stuffing
- 2 green bell pepper, large, halved
- 2 red bell peppers, large, halved
- 1 ½ cups vegetable broth
- ¾ cup quinoa
- Pinch of sea salt, add more if needed
- 1/3 tsp. cayenne pepper
- 2 Tbsp. olive oil
- 1 small onion, diced
- ¾ tsp garlic, minced
- 1 small carrot, minced
- 1 ½ celery stalks, diced
- ¾ tsp chili powder
- 1/3 cup shelled raw pumpkin seeds
- 1/3 tsp cumin
- 2 Tbsp. fresh oregano, minced
- 2 Tbsp. fresh basil, minced
- olive oil
- 1/3 cup vegetable broth

Directions:
1. Preheat the oven to 400 degrees F.
2. Pour vegetable broth into a saucepan. Put quinoa and stir well. Reduce heat and allow to simmer for 25 minutes or until the quinoa is cooked and has absorbed the liquids. Set aside.
3. Coat green and red bell peppers with olive oil. Season with salt and cayenne pepper.
4. Layer bell peppers on a baking pan, sides are facing up. Bake for 12 minutes.
5. Meanwhile, heat the olive oil in a skillet to cook the stuffing. Saute onion, garlic, carrot, celery, chili powder, pumpkin seeds, and cumin.
6. Add in cooked quinoa oregano, and basil. Mix well. Spoon mixture into the roasted pepper. Arrange the stuffed peppers in a casserole dish.

7. Pour vegetable broth around the peppers. Cover the casserole dish with aluminium foil. Bake for 20 minutes. Serve.

45. MIXED VEGGIES WITH OREGANO VINAIGRETTE

Prep Time: 10mins
Total Time: 10 mins
Servings: 2

Ingredients:

For salad
- ½ cup loosely packed radicchio, cored, stemmed, julienned, rinsed, spun-dried
- 1 cup loosely packed Romaine lettuce, julienned, rinsed, spun-dried
- 2 green Kalamata olives in brine, drained, pitted, roughly chopped
- 1 leek, root trimmed, sliced into thin diagonal slivers
- ¼ cucumber, unpeeled, halved, deseeded, sliced into thin half-moons
- 1 cup loosely packed boiled or roasted chicken, skinless, shredded, leftovers are fine, optional
- 1 cup loosely packed iceberg lettuce, julienned, rinsed, spun-dried

For dressing
- 3 Tbsp. apple cider vinegar
- 2 Tbsp. fresh oregano leaves, minced
- 1 Tbsp. extra virgin olive oil
- 1 large garlic clove, peeled, grated
- a pinch of dried oregano or oregano powder
- a pinch of dried pepper flakes, optional
- sea salt and white pepper, to taste

Directions:
1. Pour dressing ingredients into a small bottle with a tight-fitting lid. Shake well to combine.
2. Place salad ingredients into a large bowl. Drizzle in half of the dressing. Toss well to combine.
3. Spoon an equal portion of salad into plates; drizzle equal portion of remaining dressings on top. Serve.

46. ALL SEAFOOD STOCK

Prep: 15 mins
Cook: 1 hr 20 mins
Total: 1 hr 35 mins

Ingredients:
- 2 pounds fresh lobster, shrimp peelings
- 8 cups of water
- 1 carrot, chopped
- 1 Tbsp. dried chili flakes
- 2 pounds frozen fish heads and frames
- 2 large onions, halved
- 1 large celery rib, halved
- 1 garlic head, halved
- 2 Tbsp. olive oil
- 1 Tbsp. apple cider vinegar
- ¼ tsp. white pepper

Directions:
1. Preheat the oven to 220°C or 425°F. Line a deep roasting pan with aluminum foil.
2. Place fish heads and frames into a roasting dish, along with garlic, and shallots. Drizzle oil on top.
3. Place roasting pan into the middle rack of the oven. Roast fish for 25 minutes. Remove pan from oven. Transfer contents into a slow cooker, along with remaining ingredients. Secure lid. Cook broth for 8 hours.
4. Strain out and discard solids. Ladle portions into bowls. Serve with bread and salad of choice.

47. SEARED HERBED SALMON STEAK

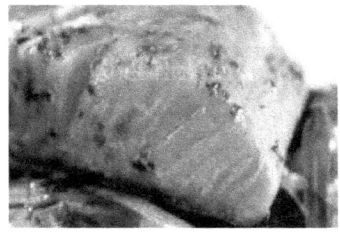

Prep Time: 10 mins

Cook Time: 5 mins
Total Time: 15 mins
Servings: 4

Ingredients:
- 1 lb salmon steak, rinsed 1/8 tsp cayenne pepper
- 1 tsp chili powder
- ½ tsp cumin
- 2 garlic cloves, minced
- 1 tablespoon olive oil
- ¾ tsp salt
- 1 tsp freshly ground black pepper

Directions:
1. Preheat the oven to 350 degrees F.
2. In a bowl, combine cayenne pepper, chili powder, cumin, salt, and black pepper. Set aside.
3. Drizzle in olive oil onto the salmon steak. Rub on both sides. Rub garlic and the prepared spice mixture. Let sit for 10 minutes.
4. After allowing the flavors to meld, prepare an ovenproof skillet. Heat the olive oil. Once hot, sear salmon for 4 minutes on both sides.
5. Transfer skillet inside the oven. Bake for 10 minutes. Serve.

48. Steamed Meatballs on Bed of Rice

Prep time: 10 mins
Cook time: 20 mins
Total time: 30 mins
Servings: 3

Ingredients:

For the beans and rice
- 1½ cups brown rice, rinsed until water runs clear, drained
- 3 cups store-bought beef or vegetable stock, low-sodium
- 1 can 15 oz. Adzuki beans or red kidney beans, rinsed, drained well
- Water, only if needed

For the meatballs
- 1 piece large egg, whisked
- 4 Tbsp. sesame oil, reserve some for greasing
- ½ cup carrots, peeled, grated, drained lightly
- ½ cup jicama, peeled, grated, drained well

- ❖ 2½ pound lean ground pork
- ❖ 1 cup frozen, peeled shrimps, thawed, drained, minced
- ❖ ½ cup chives, roots trimmed, minced
- ❖ ½ cup white onion, minced
- ❖ ¼ tsp. kosher salt
- ❖ ¼ tsp. black pepper
- ❖ 1/16 tsp. fresh ginger, peeled, grated

For dipping sauce
- ❖ 1 piece fresh bird's eye chili, stemmed, deseeded, minced
- ❖ 2 Tbsp. lemon juice, freshly squeezed
- ❖ 1 Tbsp. dark soy sauce
- ❖ ¼ cup vegan-safe light soy sauce or tamari

Directions:
1. To prepare dipping sauce: combine ingredients in a small airtight, non-reactive container. Seal lid. Shake contents of the container to mix. Set aside at room temperature until needed. This should be consumed within the week.
2. To prepare meatballs: combine ingredients in a bowl. Let meat rest for at least ten minutes before shaping.
3. Take a heaping tablespoon of meatball mix. With clean hands, roll these into a ball. Place each piece on a parchment paper-lined baking sheet. Repeat step until all meatball mix is rolled.
4. Reserve 12 pieces for immediate cooking.
5. Pack the rest in a food-grade container generously lined with saran wrap. Place strips of parchment paper in between lines and layers so these can be stacked up.
6. To prepare rice: pour ingredients into the rice cooker. The stock should reach the 3-cup line. If not, pour just enough water to reach the mark.
7. Using a pastry brush, lightly grease steaming tray with oil.
8. Place 12 pieces of meatballs into the steaming tray, spaced slightly apart, so these don't stick to each other. Secure rice cooker lid.
9. Press down on cooking button/function. Wait for the machine to automatically shift to Warm mode. Turn off the machine when ready to serve.
10. To serve: remove the steaming tray from the rice cooker. Using two spoons, carefully extract meatballs and place into individual plates.
11. Spoon equal portions of beans and rice on the side.
12. Serve with a small amount of dipping sauce on the side.

CHAPTER 3 - *ANTI-INFLAMMATORY: DINNER RECIPES*

49. HOT DUMPLING SOUP

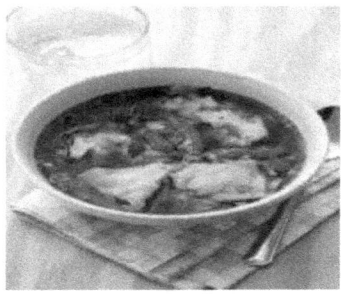

Prep Time: 1 hour
Cook Time: 15 mins
Total Time: 1 hour, 15 mins
Servings: 4

Ingredients:
- 1 pound beef bones, beef leg, oxtail
- 1 pound pork bones, pork leg, cleaned well
- cabbage leaves
- 6 cups of water
- 1 parsnip, roughly chopped
- ½ pound chicken bones and trimmings
- 3 leeks, minced
- 1 tablespoon fish sauce
- 1 carrot, roughly chopped
- 1 fresh ginger, crushed
- 1 thyme sprigs
- 1 garlic clove
- 1 white onion, quartered
- Pinch of sea salt
- Pinch of white pepper to taste

For the Filling
- 1 pound ground pork
- ¼ teaspoon garlic, grated

- ❖ ¼ teaspoon ginger, grated
- ❖ ¼ teaspoon palm sugar, crumbled
- ❖ ¼ pound fresh shrimps, minced
- ❖ ¼ cup fresh chives, minced
- ❖ 1 tablespoon rice wine vinegar
- ❖ 1 tablespoon light soy sauce
- ❖ Pinch of sea salt
- ❖ Pinch of white pepper

For the Bread
- ❖ 2 cups all-purpose flour
- ❖ ¾ cub oiled water
- ❖ ¼ cup of chilled water
- ❖ 1 tablespoon sesame oil

Directions:
1. Place soup ingredients in a large stockpot set over high heat; boil. Turn down heat to lowest setting; simmer for 4 hours. Cool completely to room temperature before straining out and discarding solids. Taste; adjust seasoning if needed.
2. Place soup in a freezer-safe container; freeze soup solid. Skim off solidified fat. Just before rolling, slice frozen, jellied soup into 6 equal-sized cubes.
3. Mix filling ingredients in a bowl; chill until ready to use.
4. Mix bread ingredients in a bowl using a wooden spoon until the dough comes together. Turn out on lightly floured surface; knead until the dough becomes elastic and no longer sticks to your hands, adding more flour as you go. Lightly grease the same mixing bowl with oil.
5. Place dough in and rest for 30 minutes, covered with a sheet of saran wrap. Divide dough into 6 equal pieces; roll into balls, tucking edges underneath to make these look seamless.
6. Half-fill steaming pot with water; set over high heat. Boil, covered; place cabbage leaves on the bottom of bamboo steaming baskets. Set aside.
7. Using a lightly floured rolling pin, flatten the dough until it is wide enough to almost fill the steaming basket. The dough should be thick in the middle, (which serves as the base of dumpling) and very thin at the edges, (which will be twisted on top.)
8. Place 1 heaping tablespoon of filling in the middle of bread, and a cube of frozen soup on top. Gather edges of bread as best as you can, pinching and sealing. Twist top slightly. Carefully place dumplings on top of cabbages in the steaming baskets; steam for 10 minutes. Remove from heat. Place entire steaming basket on a plate, with a thick-stemmed drinking straw to serve. Gently insert straw at the top of dumpling to release some heat. Cool further before consuming.

50. Artichoke Hearts Crisps

Prep Time: 10 mins
Cook Time: 30 mins
Total: 40 mins
Servings: 20

Ingredients:
- ½ lemon, sliced into wedges
- coconut oil
- 1 lb fresh artichoke hearts, quartered
- Pinch of sea salt
- Pinch of white pepper
- 1 cup almond flour
- 2 eggs, whisked
- 1 cup almond meal

Directions:
1. In a nonstick skillet set over medium heat, pour oil. Swirl pan to coat.
2. Lightly grease artichokes with salt and pepper. Dredge in almond flour, eggs, and then almond meal.
3. Slide breaded veggies into oil for 1 minute or until crisp and golden. Drain on paper towels. Serve with a wedge of lime.

51. Maple Turkey

Prep Time: 18 mins
Cook Time: 12 mins
Total Time: 30 mins
Servings: 4

Ingredients:
- 2 turkey breasts
- 2 tablespoons maple syrup
- Pinch of salt
- Pinch of pepper

Directions:
1. Season turkey breast with maple syrup, salt, and pepper.
2. Place the turkey on a greased baking sheet.
3. Bake for at least twenty minutes at 350 degrees Fahrenheit.

4. Serve with salad greens.

52. Crab Avocado Cilantro Salad

Prep Time: 15 minutes
Total Time: 15 minutes
Servings: 4

Ingredients:
- 1 avocado, cubed
- 1 pound crab meat
- 2 tablespoons mayonnaise
- 1 tablespoon lime, freshly squeezed
- Pinch of cayenne pepper
- ¼ cup fresh cilantro, chopped
- Pinch of salt
- Pinch of pepper

Directions:
1. In a bowl, mix mayonnaise, cayenne pepper, cilantro, and lime juice.
2. Season crab meat with salt and pepper. Dredge in the mayonnaise mixture.
3. Add the avocado slices. Mix well. Serve.

53. Chicken Barbeque Bake

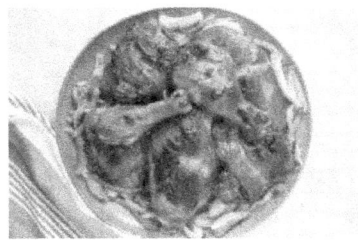

Prep Time: 10 mins
Total Time: 2 hours 5 mins
Servings: 8

Ingredients:
- 2 chicken breasts
- 4 plum tomatoes, diced
- ¼ cup barbecue sauce, low-sodium, gluten-free
- Pinch of salt
- Pinch of pepper
- ½ cup green onion, chopped
- ½ cup cheddar cheese, grated

Directions:
1. Preheat the oven to 165 degrees F.
2. Season chicken breast with salt and pepper. Place chicken in a baking dish.
3. Drizzle in barbecue sauce. Top with onion, tomatoes, and cheese.
4. Place inside the oven and bake for 30 minutes. Serve.

54. Mango Bell Pepper Salsa

Prep Time: 15 mins
Total Time: 15 mins
Servings: 3

Ingredients:
- 1 mango, chunked
- 2 pears, cored, chunked
- 1/4 cup yellow bell pepper, finely chopped
- 1/4 cup red bell pepper, finely chopped
- ¼ cup red onion, finely chopped
- 2 tsp. olive oil
- 3 tbsp. fresh cilantro, chopped
- 1 jalapeño pepper, finely chopped
- Pinch of salt
- 1 tbsp. lime juice

Directions:
1. Mix mango, red onion, pears, yellow bell pepper, red bell pepper, olive oil, cilantro, jalapeño pepper, salt, and lime juice in a bowl. Mix well until all ingredients are well combined. Wrap bowl.
2. Pace inside the refrigerator. Serve asneeded.

55. Buttered Cauliflower Mash

Prep Time: 15 Mins
Cook Time: 15 Mins
Total Time: 30 mins
Servings: 6

Ingredients:
- 1 cup cauliflower florets
- ¼ cup sour cream
- 2 tbsp. salted butter
- Pinch of pepper

Directions:
1. Steam cauliflower florets for 5 minutes or until soft.
2. Process steamed florets in a food processor.
3. Add in butter and sour cream. Process again until all ingredients are well combined. Serve.

56. Salmon and Pickle Salad

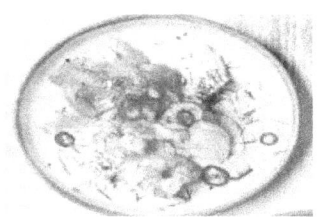

Prep: 40 mins
Total Time: 40 mins
Serves 4 - 6

Ingredients:
- 1 can salmon, drained
- 1/3 cup of pickle relish
- ¼ cup mayonnaise
- 1 cup onion, minced
- 1 celery, minced
- Fresh herbs of choice

Directions:
1. In a salad bowl, put together salmon, mayonnaise, onion, pickle relish, celery, and fresh herbs of choice.
2. Mix all the ingredients until well combined. Serve.

57. GARLIC LEAN PORK

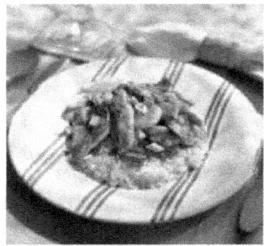

Prep Time: 25 Mins
Cook Time: 9 Mins
Total Time: 24 mins
Servings: 4

Ingredients:
- 3 tablespoons of soy sauce
- Pinch of pepper
- Pinch of salt
- Olive oil
- 2 slices of a lean pork chop
- Cumin
- 5 cloves of minced garlic

Directions:
1. In a zip lock bag, combine
2. Place the soy sauce, pepper, salt, pork chops, cumin, and garlic in a zip bag and refrigerate overnight.
3. The next day, heat the oil in a pan and cook the pork chops for three to seven minutes per side or until well done.
4. Serve with fresh fruits.

58. OLIVES AND EGGS ROLLUPS

Prep Time: 10 mins
Total Time: 5 mins
Servings: 4

Ingredients:
- 1 egg
- 5 kalamata olives, pitted
- ½ cup sun-dried tomatoes in oil
- 1/8 tsp. salt
- 1/8 tsp. pepper
- 2 tbsp. olive oil, divided
- 1/8 tsp. parsley flakes
- 1/8 tsp. red chili flakes

Directions:
1. In a bowl, mix egg, salt, pepper, and olive oil. Whisk the mixture until foamy.
2. Heat a skillet. Pour olive oil. Pour the egg mixture, making sure to spread evenly in the pan forming a thin layer.
3. Cook egg for 3 minutes on both sides. Remove and transfer to a plate.
4. Meanwhile, in a food processor, put together tomatoes, olives, parsley, and chili flakes. Process until the mixture is well blended.
5. Spread mixture on top of the frittata.
6. Roll frittata and cut into bite-sized pieces. Serve.

59. ASPARAGUS AND PEPPERS TERRINE

Prep Time: 20 mins
Cook Time: 20 mins
Total Time: 40 mins
Servings: 4

Ingredients:
- 1 tbsp. olive oil
- 1 red pepper, quartered
- 2 carrots, sliced diagonally
- 1 green pepper, quartered
- ¾ cup full soft cheese
- 1 tbsp. fresh parsley, chopped
- 4 fresh green asparagus stalks

- 1 cup almond milk, unsweetened
- ¼ cup double cream
- 4 eggs, beaten
- Pinch of salt
- Pinch of ground black pepper
- Salad leaves
- 2 tomatoes, halved
- ½ cucumber, sliced

Directions:
1. Preheat the oven to 350 degrees F. Grease a loaf tin.
2. Put the pepper quarters on a grill rack. Cook for 4 minutes on both sides or until the skins have charred. Transfer to a plate. Cover with kitchen paper. Allow cooling.
3. Meanwhile, in a pan. Pour water. Cook carrots and asparagus for 3 minutes or until tender. Drain with kitchen paper. Peel off skins of pepper.
4. In a bowl, put together eggs, milk, soft cheese, and cream. Stir well. Season with salt and pepper.
5. Arrange vegetables on the loaf tin. Spoon cheese mixture over the veggies. Layer vegetables and cheese mixture and then layer the pepper on top.
6. Cover tin with foil. Pour in boiling water of the roasting tin.
7. Bake for 45 minutes. Remove from the roasting tin and allow cooling. Liftoff the lining paper. Slice terrine.
8. Serve with salad leaves, tomatoes, and cucumber.

60. MUSHROOMS AND BABY ONIONS

Prep Time: 38 Mins
Cook Time: 5 mins
Total Time: 43 Mins
Serving: 4

Ingredients:
- 2 carrots, peeled, diced
- 2 baby onions, tops and roots trimmed
- 3 tbsp. olive oil
- ½ cup dry white wine
- 1 tsp. coriander seeds, lightly crushed
- 2 bay leaves
- Dash of cayenne pepper
- 1 garlic clove, crushed

- 3 tomatoes, quartered
- Pinch of salt
- Pinch of pepper
- 3 tbsp. fresh parsley, chopped, for garnish

Directions:
1. Heat the olive oil in a pan. Add onions and carrots. Cool for 15 minutes or until the vegetables have turned light brown.
2. Pour white wine. Garlic, coriander seeds, mushrooms, bay leaves, and tomatoes. Cook for 20 minutes or until the vegetables are tender and the sauce thickens.
3. Transfer to a plate. Allow cooling. You may also choose to chill before serving. Drizzle in olive oil. Sprinkle parsley. Serve.

61. ARTICHOKE SOUP

Prep time: 25 mins
Cook time: 1 hour, 20 mins
Servings: 8

Ingredients:
- 2 tbsp. olive oil
- 1 garlic clove, chopped
- 1 onion, chopped
- 1 celery stick, chopped
- 4 cups vegetable stock
- 1 ½ lb. artichokes, chopped
- 2 cups almond milk
- Pinch of salt, add more if needed
- Pinch of pepper, add more if needed

Directions:
1. Heat the olive oil in a large saucepan. Sauté garlic, onion, and celery. Stir occasionally for 5 minutes.
2. Pour vegetable stock. Season mixture with salt and pepper. Bring mixture to a boil.
3. Reduce heat. Allow to simmer for 20 minutes or until the artichokes are tender. Let the soup cool before transferring in a blender.
4. Once cooled, process until smooth and creamy.
5. Return soup in the saucepan. Pour milk. Let it simmer for 2 minutes.
6. Ladle into bowls. Adjust taste if needed. Serve.

62. Courgettes and Peppers with Cashew Nuts

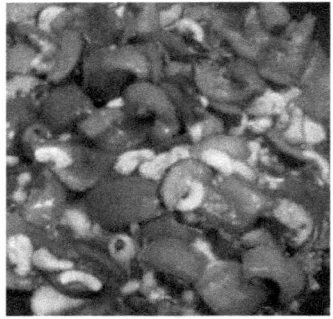

Prep time: 5 mins
Cook time: 35 mins
Total time: 40 mins
Servings: 4

Ingredients:
- 2 carrots, cut into matchsticks
- 1 red pepper, cut into matchsticks
- 1 green pepper, cut into matchsticks
- 2 courgettes, cut into matchsticks
- Bunch of spring onions, chopped
- 1 tbsp. extra virgin olive oil
- 4 curry leaves
- ½ tsp. white cumin seeds
- 3 red chilies, dried
- 10 cashew nuts
- 1 tsp. salt
- 2 tbsp. lemon juice
- Fresh mint leaves, for garnish

Directions:
1. Heat the olive oil in a pan. Stir fry curry leaves, dried chilies, and cumin seeds for 2 minutes.
2. Add in cashew nuts, carrots, and courgettes. Cook for 4 minutes or until the vegetables are tender.
3. Transfer to a serving dish. Discard dried chilies. Serve.

63. Salmon with Broccoli and Sweet Potato

Prep Time: 5mins
Cook Time: 20 mins
Total Time: 25 mins
Servings: 4

Ingredients:
- 4 salmon fillets
- 3 red sweet potatoes
- 1 pound Chinese broccoli
- 1 tsp. Chinese mustard
- Pinch of salt
- 1 cup balsamic vinegar
- 2 teaspoons yellow mustard seeds
- 2 tablespoons vegetable oil, divided
- 1 ½ tsp gluten-free soy sauce

Directions:
1. Preheat the oven to 400 degrees °F.
2. Prepare sweet potato by wrapping them individually in a foil.
3. In a baking pan, lay the wrapped sweet potatoes and roast for 1 hour. Allow cooling before peeling them.
4. Run peeled sweet potatoes in a blender until smooth. Transfer into a heating bowl.
5. Add mustard. Season with salt. Put inside the refrigerator for 1 hour.
6. Meanwhile, in a saucepan, pour vinegar. Let it boil until reduced. Tip in soy sauce. Remove from heat.
7. In a pot, pour water and salt. Boil the broccoli for 3 minutes or until tender but crisp.
8. In a spice mill, process the mustard seeds until it is coarsely ground.
9. Get the fish and season it with salt and pepper. Season it with mustard seeds.
10. In a skillet, heat the oil. Cook the fish, mustard side down. Do so until it is brown but tender in the centre. Get the pureed sweet potatoes and reheat it.
11. In another skillet, heat the oil. Sauté broccoli. Season with salt and pepper.
12. To serve, place the broccoli, puree, and the fish side by side. Drizzle with balsamic vinegar.

64. Turkey Salad

Prep Time: 5 mins
Total Time: 5 mins
Servings: 2

Ingredients:
- 1 ½ pound of sliced turkey breast
- ¾ cups of red grapes
- 4 stalks of celery
- 1/3 cup of pistachio nuts
- Salt
- Pepper
- 1/3 cup of light mayonnaise

Directions:
1. In a bowl, put together turkey, celery, grapes, pistachios, and mayonnaise. Season with salt and pepper.
2. Chill in the refrigerator for 30 minutes. Serve.

65. Zucchini Endive Soup

Prep Time: 10 mins
Cook Time: 20 mins
Total Time: 30 mins
Servings : 4

Ingredients:
- 1 tsp olive oil
- 1 cup zucchini, shredded
- 1 cup curly endive, chopped
- ½ cup chopped onion
- ½ cup of water
- 1 cup vegetable broth
- 2 tablespoons fresh dill, chopped
- ½ tsp honey
- ½ tablespoon green onion, chopped

Directions:
1. Place a saucepan over medium heat. Add oil. Swirl to coat.
2. Stir in onion and sauté for 3 minutes or until tender. Pour water and broth. Bring to a boil.

3. Stir zucchini and dill. Boil again. Reduce to a simmer for 3 minutes.
4. Pour lemon juice, honey, endive, salt, and pepper. Simmer for 3 minutes, uncovered. Scatter green onions. Serve.

66. UNSALTED VEGETABLE BROTH

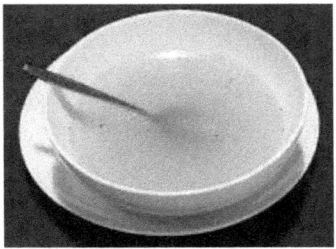

Prep Time: 10 mins
Cook Time: 30 mins
Total Time: 40 mins
Servings: 16

Ingredients:
- 12 cups water
- 1 cup squash, cubed
- Broccoli and cauliflower stems
- 2 pieces celery ribs, chopped
- 2 pieces large garlic cloves, crushed
- 1 piece large carrot, roughly chopped
- 1 piece large white onion, peeled, quartered
- 2 Tbsp. fresh red peppercorns
- Corn cob
- Leftover frozen vegetables, store-bought
- Leftover seeds, unseasoned
- Mushroom trimmings
- Peels from carrots, potatoes, daikon, turnip, parsnips, radish, etc.
- Wilted herbs

Directions:
1. Pour ingredients in the large Dutch oven set over a high flame. Stir gently. Secure lid.
2. Cook broth for 20 minutes or until most of the vegetables is soft.
3. Strain out and discard solids.
4. Ladle portions into bowls. Serve with bread and salad of choice.

67. Spiced Mussel Broth

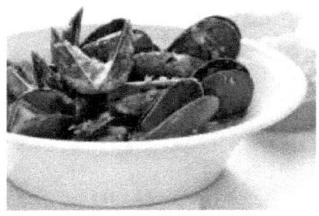

Prep Time: 15mins
Cook Time: 15 mins
Total Time: 30 mins
Servings: 4

Ingredients:

- 4 ½ lb. black mussels, cleaned
- 7 spring onions, sliced thinly
- 3 fresh red chilies, halved
- 9 kaffir lime leaves, crushed
- 3 garlic cloves, crushed
- 4 ½ cups chicken broth
- 3 Tbsp. sliced ginger
- 3 Tbsp. coriander leaves, chopped
- 1 ½ Tbsp. cooking oil

Directions:

1. Place a wok over medium flame and add the oil. Sauté the spring onion and garlic until tender.
2. Add the lemongrass, chili, lime leaves, galangal, 4 ½ cups of water, and broth.
3. Stir in the mussels, cover, and boil for 8 minutes or until the mussels open. Remove unopened mussels.
4. Add half the coriander and stir. Divide the broth and mussels into individual bowls. Top with the reserved coriander.

68. Hot Kiwi, Mango, Berries Salad

Prep Time: 45 mins
Total Time: 45 mins
Servings: 4

Ingredients:
- 1 kiwi fruit, quartered
- 1 ripe mango, cubed
- 1 strawberry, quartered
- ½ cup fresh blueberries

For the Dressing
- 1 tablespoon lime juice, freshly squeezed
- ⅛ teaspoon maple syrup
- ⅛ teaspoon chili powder

Directions:
1. Place dressing ingredients into a small bottle with a tight-fitting lid. Seal and shake the bottle until salt dissolves.
2. Place salad ingredients into a bowl; drizzle in dressing. Toss to combine.
3. Place equal portions into bowls. Serve immediately.

69. All Mushroom Soup

Prep Time: 10 mins
Cook Time: 25 mins
Total Time: 35 mins
Servings: 4

Ingredients:
- 2½ cups vegetable stock, unsalted
- 2 Tbsp. olive oil
- 1 garlic clove, minced
- 1 onion, minced
- 1 poblano chili, diced
- 1 jalapeño pepper, diced
- 1 red bell pepper, diced
- 1 winter squash, cubed
- 1 zucchini, cubed
- 1 can straw mushrooms, halved

- ❖ 1 can whole button mushrooms, halved
- ❖ ½ tsp. coriander powder

Directions:
1. Pour olive oil into a Dutch oven set over medium heat.
2. Add in and stir fry garlic and onions until limp and aromatic.
3. Stir in Anaheim, jalapeño, and red bell peppers. Cook these for 15 minutes, stirring often.
4. Pour in unsalted vegetable stock along with acorn and yellow squash. Season with coriander, salt, and pepper. Bring stock to a rolling boil. Secure lid. Turn down heat to the lowest setting. Let the soup simmer for 10 to 15 minutes or until squashes are fork-tender.
5. Stir in remaining ingredients. Turn off heat when zucchini is crisp-tender. This would take another 5 to 10 minutes. Taste. Adjust seasoning if needed.
6. Ladle the desired amount into a bowl. Cool slightly before serving.

70. TUNA SALAD WRAPPED IN LETTUCE

Ingredients:
- ❖ 6 leaves Romaine lettuce
- ❖ 1 onion, sliced thinly

For the filling
- ❖ 1 can tuna chunks in water, drained
- ❖ 1 Tbsp. English mustard
- ❖ 1 Tbsp. tuna brine
- ❖ 1 Tbsp. Greek yoghurt
- ❖ Dash of Spanish paprika
- ❖ Dash of curry powder
- ❖ 1 green chili, minced

Directions:
1. For the onion pickle, using your fingers, mash onion slices and salt in a small bowl. Set aside for 15 minutes, uncovered.
2. After 15 minutes, rinse onions under running water. Drain well using a strainer. Set aside until ready to use.
3. For the tuna filling, combine all ingredients in a large bowl. Taste. Adjust seasoning, if needed. Chill well before using.
4. To assemble, spread a generous teaspoon of filling along the inner spine of each lettuce leaf. Serve immediately.

71. FISH EGG ROLLS

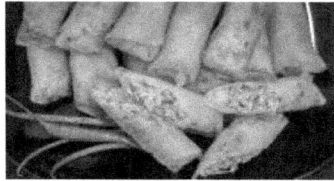

Prep Time: 12 mins
Cook Time: 6 mins
Total Time: 18 mins
Servings: 4

Ingredients:
- 8 pieces spring roll wrappers, large
- oil, for deep frying
- water, for sealing

Filling
- 8 pieces asparagus
- 2 tablespoons fresh chives, minced
- 2 tablespoons fresh cilantro, minced
- ½ tablespoons light soy sauce
- 1 can slice bamboo shoots, drained
- ½ pound halibut fillets
- Dash of white pepper

Dipping sauce
- 4 tablespoons packed palm sugar, crumbled
- 2 tablespoons fish sauce
- 2 tablespoons tomato catsup
- ½ teaspoon white pepper
- ⅛ cup of rice wine vinegar
- Pinch of sea salt to taste

Directions:
1. Combine dipping sauce ingredients in a bowl. Stir until sugar dissolves. Taste; adjust seasoning if needed.
2. Season halibut fillets with soy sauce and white pepper. Place a fillet on 1 corner of spring roll wrapper. Add equal portions of asparagus, bamboo shoots, chives, and cilantro on top. Roll tightly, folding in edges, and sealing with water. Set aside. Repeat step for remaining ingredients.

3. Half-fill deep fryer with oil set at medium heat; wait for the oil to become slightly smoky before sliding in spring rolls. Cook only until spring rolls turn golden brown, 5 to 7 minutes. Transfer cooked spring rolls to a plate lined with paper towels. Place 2 spring rolls on a plate; serve with dipping sauce on the side.

72. VEGGIE ROLLS

Prep Time25 mins
Total Time25 mins
Servings: 4

Ingredients:
- 8 pieces spring roll wrappers
- oil, for deep frying
- water, for sealing

Filling
- 1 tablespoon coconut oil
- 1 tablespoon chicken concentrate
- 1 garlic clove, minced
- 1 shallot, julienned
- 1 cup bean sprouts
- ¼ cup carrots, julienned
- ¼ cup potato, julienned
- ¼ cup squash, julienned
- ¼ cup sweet potato, julienned
- ¼ cup cooked chicken, shredded
- ½ cup of water
- Pinch of sea salt
- Pinch of black pepper

Dipping sauce
- 4 tablespoons palm sugar, crumbled
- 4 tablespoons fish sauce
- 4 tablespoons of rice wine vinegar
- 1 tablespoon grated garlic
- 1 tablespoon grated ginger
- 1 piece banana chili, minced
- 1 piece bird's eye chili, minced
- Pinch of black pepper

Directions:

1. Combine dipping sauce ingredients in a bowl. Stir until sugar dissolves. Taste; adjust seasoning if needed. Set aside.
2. To make spring rolls: pour coconut oil into large wok set over medium heat. Sauté garlic and shallot until limp and transparent; except for bean sprouts, add in remaining filling ingredients. Cook until root crops are fork-tender. Toss in bean sprouts; stir. Turn off the heat immediately. Allow filling to cool completely to room temperature before rolling.
3. Add equal portions of vegetable filling into spring roll paper; roll tightly, tucking in the edges and sealing with water. Set aside. Repeat step for remaining filling/wrapper.
4. Half-fill deep fryer with cooking oil set at medium heat; wait for the oil to become slightly smoky before sliding in spring rolls. Cook only until spring rolls turn golden brown, about 7 minutes. Transfer cooked pieces on a plate lined with paper towels. Place 2 spring rolls on a plate; serve with dipping sauce on the side.

73. CABBAGE AND FISH EGG ROLLS

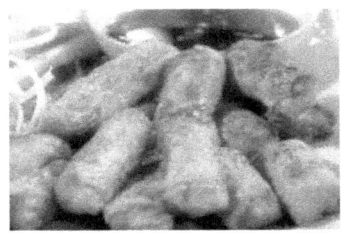

Prep Time: 25 mins
Cook Time: 15 mins
Total Time: 40 mins
Servings: 4

Ingredients:

Filling

- 1 tablespoon sesame oil
- 1 tablespoon light soy sauce
- ½ tablespoon oyster sauce
- 1 cup cabbage, julienned
- ¼ cupcarrot, minced
- ¼ cup shallot, minced

- ¼ cup of water
- ¼ teaspoons ginger, grated
- ½ pound white fish fillets, diced
- 8 pieces spring roll wrappers
- oil, for deep frying
- water, for sealing

Dipping sauce
- 2 drops sesame oil
- ¼ cup mayonnaise
- ¼ tablespoon lemon juice, freshly squeezed
- ¼ tablespoon light soy sauce
- ¼ tablespoon sesame seeds, toasted
- ¼ teaspoon garlic, grated
- Pinch of sea salt
- Pinch of black pepper

Directions:
1. Mix dipping sauce ingredients in a bowl until salt dissolves. Taste; adjust seasoning if needed.
2. To make the filling: pour sesame oil into non-stick wok set over medium heat. Sauté ginger and shallot until limp and aromatic; add in carrots, soy sauce and water. Stir-fry until carrots are fork-tender.
3. Add remaining ingredients into wok. Cook only until fish turns transparent. Turn off heat; cool before rolling. Add equal portions of filling into spring roll paper; roll tightly, tucking in the edges and sealing with water. Set aside. Repeat step for remaining filling.
4. Half-fill deep fryer with cooking oil set at medium heat; wait for the oil to become slightly smoky before sliding in spring rolls. Cook only until spring rolls turn golden brown, about 5 minutes. Transfer cooked spring rolls to a plate lined with paper towels. Place 2 spring rolls on a plate; serve with dipping sauce on the side.

74. PORK FILLET NOODLES

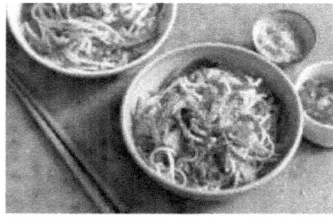

Prep Time: 5 mins
Cook Time: 15 mins
Total Time: 20 mins
Serves 4

Ingredients:
- 8 oz egg noodles
- 8 oz cooked pork fillet
- 2 tablespoons light soy sauce
- 2 spring onions, shredded
- 5 tablespoons vegetable oil
- ½ teaspoon salt
- ½ teaspoon sugar

Directions:
1. Cook the noodles in boiling water. Strain well.
2. Slice meat into thin slices. Top and tail the beans.
3. Heat the oil in a wok. Add noodle and soy sauce. Stir-fry for 3 minutes. Remove and transfer to a serving dish.
4. Heat the remaining oil. Tip in salt, sugar, and soy sauce. Stir well. Pour a little stock.
5. Pour seafood mixture on top of the noodles. Drizzle sesame oil. Garnish with spring onions.

75. CHICKEN NOODLE SOUP

Prep Time 15 mins
Cook Time 15 mins
Total Time 30 mins
Servings: 6

Ingredients:
- 8 oz cooked chicken breasts
- 8 oz egg noodles
- 5 tablespoons vegetable oil
- 2 tablespoons light soy sauce
- ½ teaspoon salt
- ½ teaspoon sugar
- 2 spring onions, shredded

Directions:
1. Cook the noodles in boiling water. Strain well.
2. Slice meat into thin slices. Top and tail the beans.
3. Heat the oil in a wok. Add noodle and soy sauce. Stir-fry for 3 minutes. Remove and transfer to a serving dish.

4. Heat the remaining oil. Tip in salt, sugar, and soy sauce. Stir well. Pour a little stock.
5. Pour seafood mixture on top of the noodles. Drizzle sesame oil. Garnish with spring onions.

76. ZUCCHINI, KALE, AND SHRIMP NOODLES

Prep Time: 5 mins
Cook Time: 10 mins
Total Time: 15 mins
Servings: 2

Ingredients:
- 3 tablespoons olive oil
- ¾ tablespoon five-spice powder
- 1 pound fresh shrimps, deveined
- ½ pound fresh kale leaves, shredded
- Pinch of sea salt
- Pinch of black pepper

Salad
- 3 tablespoons sesame oil
- 1 thumb-sized ginger, julienned
- 1 carrot, julienned
- 1 white onion, julienned
- 1 zucchini, processed into long spaghetti noodle
- 1 lime, sliced into wedges
- ¼ cup rice wine vinegar

Directions:
1. Pour 2 tablespoons of olive oil into wok set over high heat. Sauté shrimps with salt, five-spice powder and pepper; cook until shrimps turn coral. Transfer cooked pieces into a salad bowl.
2. Pour remaining olive oil into the same wok; add in kale leaves and a small pinch of salt. Cook until leaves wilt. Place kale leaves on top of shrimps; cool before adding in remaining ingredients.
3. Place remaining ingredients into a salad bowl. Toss well to combine; spoon equal portions into plates. Taste; adjust seasoning if needed. Serve.

77. RICE AND PRAWN NOODLES

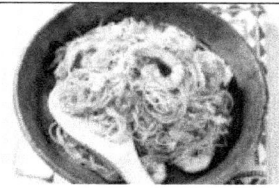

Prep Time: 15 mins
Cook Time: 10 mins
Total Time: 25 mins
Servings: 4

Ingredients:
- 2 cups rice vermicelli
- 4 oz cooked chicken
- 2 oz frozen prawns, thawed
- 4 tablespoons vegetable oil
- 1 onion, shredded
- 1 teaspoon salt
- 1 tablespoon curry powder
- 2 tablespoons light soy sauce
- 2 green or red chili peppers
- 2 spring onions, shredded

Directions:
1. Soak rice vermicelli in boiling water for 10 minutes. Rinse in cold water.
2. Slice pork meat thinly. Dry prawns in paper towel.
3. Heat oil in a wok. Stir fry onion for 2 minutes.
4. Add noodles, meat, and prawns. Stir for 3 minutes.
5. Tip in curry powder, soy sauce, chili peppers, and spring onions. Stir fry for 1 minute. Serve.

78. RICE BEEF, AND PRAWNS NOODLES

Prep Time: 5 mins
Cook Time: 15 mins
Total Time: 20 mins
Servings: 4

Ingredients:
- ❖ 2 cups rice vermicelli
- ❖ 4 oz cooked beef
- ❖ 2 oz frozen prawns, thawed
- ❖ 4 tablespoons vegetable oil
- ❖ 1 onion, shredded
- ❖ 2 cups bean sprouts
- ❖ 1 teaspoon salt
- ❖ 1 tablespoon curry powder
- ❖ 2 tablespoons light soy sauce
- ❖ 2 green or red chili peppers
- ❖ 2 spring onions, shredded

Directions:
1. Soak rice vermicelli in boiling water for 10 minutes. Rinse in cold water.
2. Slice beef meat thinly. Dry prawns in paper towel.
3. Heat oil in a wok. Stir fry onion for 2 minutes.
4. Add noodles, beef, and prawns. Stir for 3 minutes.
5. Tip in curry powder, soy sauce, chili peppers, and spring onions. Stir fry for 1 minute. Serve.

79. RICE AND CHICKEN NOODLES

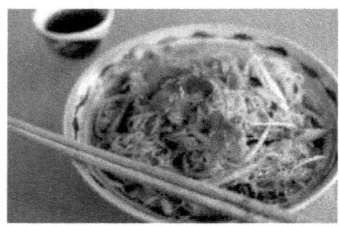

Prep Time: 10 mins
Cook Time: 20 mins
Total Time: 30 mins
Servings: 2

Ingredients:
- ❖ 2 cups rice vermicelli
- ❖ 4 oz cooked chicken
- ❖ 2 oz frozen prawns, thawed
- ❖ 4 tablespoons vegetable oil
- ❖ 1 onion, shredded

- ❖ 2 cups bean sprouts
- ❖ 1 teaspoon salt
- ❖ 1 tablespoon curry powder
- ❖ 2 tablespoons light soy sauce
- ❖ 2 green or red chili peppers
- ❖ 2 spring onions, shredded

Directions:
1. Soak rice vermicelli in boiling water for 10 minutes. Rinse in cold water.
2. Slice chicken meat thinly. Dry prawns in paper towel.
3. Heat oil in a wok. Stir fry onion and beans for 2 minutes.
4. Add noodles, chicken, and prawns. Stir for 3 minutes.
5. Tip in curry powder, soy sauce, chili peppers, and spring onions. Stir fry for 1 minute. Serve.

80. EGG AND MUSHROOMS BAKE

Prep time: 10 mins
Cook time: 20 mins
Total time: 30 mins
Servings: 4

Ingredients:
- ❖ 2 cups wild mushrooms, finely chopped
- ❖ 3 tbsp. butter
- ❖ 2 onions, finely chopped
- ❖ 1 garlic clove, finely chopped
- ❖ 2 tbsp. crème Fraiche
- ❖ 1 tbsp. lemon juice
- ❖ 1 tsp. fresh tarragon, chopped
- ❖ 2 tbsp. fresh chives snipped, reserve some for garnish
- ❖ 5 eggs
- ❖ Pinch of salt
- ❖ Pinch of pepper

Directions:
1. Preheat the oven to 375 degrees F.
2. Meanwhile, heat the butter in a pan. Cook the onions and garlic for 3 minutes or until browned and softened.
3. Add in mushrooms. Stir frequently until the mushrooms lose its moisture, and the colour is starting to turn into brown.
4. Tip in tarragon and lemon juice. Put half tablespoon of the crème Fraiche and chives. Season with salt and pepper.

5. Distribute mushroom mixture into ramekins. Sprinkle chives.
6. Break an egg into each ramekin. Place inside the oven and bake for 15 minutes or until the eggs are set.
7. Garnish with chives. Serve.

81. Spinach, Artichoke, and Pumpkin Seeds Casserole

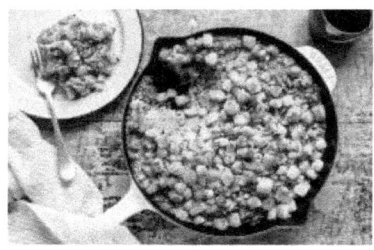

Prep Time: 5 mins
Cook Time: 35 mins
Total Time: 40 mins
Servings: 6

Ingredients:
- 2 tbsp. olive oil
- ½ cup fresh spinach leaves
- 3 turnips, sliced
- 3 leeks, sliced
- 1 red bell pepper, sliced
- ½ cup artichoke hearts
- 4 tbsp. pumpkin seeds
- Pinch of salt
- Pinch of ground black pepper

Directions:
1. Preheat the oven to 350 degrees F. Pour olive oil unto the casserole.
2. Place leeks, turnips, spinach, artichoke hearts, and red bell pepper in the saucepan.
3. Cover the casserole. Place inside the microwave oven. Bake for 30 minutes or until the turnips have softened.
4. Sprinkle pumpkin seeds. Season with salt and pepper. Serve.

82. Chicken Salad with Cabbage and Lettuce

Prep time: 30 mins
Cook time: 30 mins
Total time: 1 hour
Servings: 4

Ingredients:

For the Vinaigrette
- 1 garlic clove, grated
- 1 teaspoon ginger, grated
- 1 teaspoon soy sauce
- 1 tablespoon sesame oil
- ¼ tablespoon palm crumble
- ¼ cuprice wine vinegar

For the Salad
- 2 heads Romaine lettuce, torn to bite-sized pieces
- 2 cups roasted chicken, diced
- ½ cup red cabbage, julienned
- ¼ cup almond slivers, toasted
- ¼ cup carrots, grated
- ¼ cup edamame, cooked
- 1 leek, minced
- 1 teaspoon sesame seeds, toasted, for garnish

Directions:
1. Whisk vinaigrette ingredients in a bowl until solids dissolve. Taste; adjust seasoning if needed. Set aside.
2. Place salad ingredients in a bowl; drizzle half of the vinaigrette on top. Toss well to combine. Place equal portions of salad into plates. Drizzle in remaining vinaigrette, and garnish with toasted sesame seeds. Serve.

83. Fish Stock with Ginger

Prep Time: 15 mins
Cook Time: 20 mins
Total Time: 35 mins
Servings: 4

Ingredients:
- 8 cups of water
- ⅛ cup garlic, minced
- 4 pounds of fish frames
- 4 leeks, roughly chopped
- 2 carrots, roughly chopped
- 2 shallots, julienned
- 1 thumb-sized ginger, crushed
- 2 Tbsp. coconut oil
- 1 Tbsp. coconut vinegar

Directions:
1. Pour olive oil, garlic, ginger, onion, and white parts of leeks into large Dutch oven set over a high flame. Sauté for 3 to 5 minutes or until onions are limp and transparent.
2. Pour in remaining ingredients. Carefully stir.
3. Bring stock to a rolling boil. Turn down heat to the lowest flame. Secure lid.
4. Simmer stock for 25 minutes. Turn off heat.
5. Strain out and discard solids. Cool slightly.
6. Ladle portions into bowls. Serve with bread and salad of choice.

84. CUCUMBER, CORN, AND BELL PEPPER SALAD

Prep Time 10 mins
Cook Time: 15 mins
Total Time: 25 mins
Servings: 4

Ingredients:
- 1 cucumber, chopped
- 1 can whole kernel corn, drained
- 1 green bell pepper, chopped
- 1 red bell pepper, chopped
- 2 tablespoons red wine vinegar
- 1 tablespoon red pepper flakes, crushed
- 1/2 teaspoon garlic, minced
- 1/2 teaspoon cumin
- 1/4 teaspoon dried cilantro

Directions:
1. Combine cucumber, corn, green bell pepper, red bell pepper, and red wine vinegar in a large salad bowl.
2. Season with crushed red pepper flakes, garlic, cumin, and cilantro.
3. Cover the bowl and place inside the fridge for 30 minutes or until ready to serve.

85. ASIAN CHICKEN SALAD

Prep time: 2 hours 15 mins
Cook time: 10 mins
Total time: 2 hours 25 mins
Servings: 4

Ingredients:

For the salad
- 3 cups cooked chicken, shredded
- ¼ cup raw cashew nuts, roasted
- 1 handful cilantro leaves, torn
- 1 can crushed pineapple
- 1 carrot, julienned
- 1 avocado, cubed
- ½ red bell pepper, julienned
- ½ head purple cabbage, shredded
- ½ head green cabbage, shredded
- 12 stalks chives, minced

For the dressing
- ½ cup peanut butter, organic
- 3 Tbsp. boiled water
- 2 Tbsp. rice wine vinegar
- 2 Tbsp. stevia
- ¼ tsp. sesame oil

Directions:
1. For the dressing, combine all ingredients in a small mixing bowl. Whisk well.
2. For the salad, combine all ingredients into a large salad bowl. Drizzle 2 tablespoons of dressings on top. Toss salad well to combine. Divide into 4 equal portions.
3. To serve, plate one portion of salad on a plate. Drizzle more dressing, if desired. Serve immediately.

86. Mushroom Curry

Prep Time: 10 mins
Cook Time: 45 mins
Total Time: 55 mins
Servings: 4

Ingredients:
- 2 tbsp. olive oil
- ½ tsp. cumin seeds
- ¼ tsp. black peppercorns
- 3 green cardamom pods
- ¼ tsp. ground turmeric
- 1 onion, finely chopped
- 1 tsp. ground cumin
- 1 tsp. ground coriander
- ½ tsp. garam masala
- 1 fresh green chili, finely chopped
- 2 garlic cloves, crushed
- 1 fresh root ginger, grated
- 1 can tomatoes, chopped
- ¼ tsp salt
- 4 cups button mushrooms, halved
- Fresh coriander, chopped, for garnish

Directions:
1. In a large saucepan, heat the olive oil set over low heat. Add cardamom pods, cumin seeds, peppercorns, and turmeric. Cook for 3 minutes.
2. Stir in onions, ground coriander, cumin, and garam masala. Cook for 4 minutes.
3. Tip in the garlic, ginger, and chili. Continue stirring and cook for 3 minutes. This will prevent the spices from sticking to the pan.
4. Pour tomatoes. Season with salt and pepper. Let the mixture simmer for 5 minutes.
5. Tip in mushrooms. Cover the pan and allow simmering for up to 10 minutes. Discard cardamom pods. Garnish with coriander. Serve.

87. Baked Stuffed Meatballs

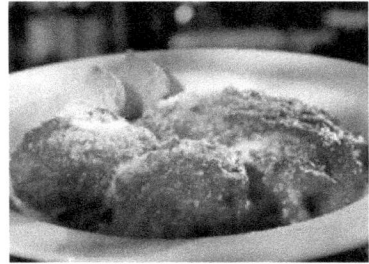

Prep Time: 20 min
Cook Time: 45 min
Total Time: 1 hr 5 mins
Servings: 4

Ingredients:
- sourdough rolls, about 3-inches long, sliced lengthwise, warmed through
- parsley leaves, chopped
- Mozzarella cheese

Marinara Sauce
- ½ Tbsp. olive oil
- 1 white onion, minced
- 2 garlic cloves, minced
- 1 can tomato puree
- ¼ Tbsp. dried red pepper, crushed
- ⅛ tsp. white pepper
- ¼ cup water
- ¼ Tbsp. dried basil

Meatballs
- 1½ pounds lean ground beef
- ¼ cup old-fashioned oats
- Pinch of salt
- Pinch of pepper
- 2 egg, whisked until frothy

Directions:
1. Preheat the oven to 400°F. Line a roasting pan with aluminium foil.
2. For the marinara sauce, pour olive oil into a large saucepan. Sauté onion and garlic for 3 minutes or until limp and transparent.

3. Add in tomato puree, dried red pepper, brown sugar, white pepper, water, and dried basil. Bring to a soft boil.
4. Reduce the heat and allow to simmer for 15 minutes with the lid on.
5. For the meatballs, put together lean ground beef, old-fashioned oats, salt, pepper, and eggs in a large bowl. Mix. Cover with saran wrap. Set aside for 10 minutes. Stir again.
6. Divide mixture into equal portions. Roll into small balls. Place balls into the roasting pan. Pour marinara sauce all over.
7. Place roasting pan in the middle rack of the oven. Cook for 10 minutes.
8. Reduce the heat to 300°F. Cook for another 25 minutes. Remove from the oven. Let sit for a few minutes.
9. To serve, stuff 3 meatballs in sourdough rolls. Drizzle in marinara sauce on top. Scatter parsley and mozzarella cheese.

88. MELON AND WATERMELON SALAD

Prep Time: 2 mins
Total Time: 2 mins
Servings: 4

Ingredients:
- 12 scoops yellow-fleshed watermelon, preferably seedless
- 12 scoops red-fleshed watermelon, preferably seedless
- 12 scoops sugar melon
- 6 scoops cantaloupe
- 6 scoops honeydew melon

Directions:
1. Combine fruits in a freezer safe container.
2. Place the container in the deep freeze for at least 10 minutes before serving; spoon equal portions into bowls. Serve.

89. BEEF MUSHROOM SOUP

Prep Time: 10 mins
Cook Time: 20 mins
Total Time: 30 min.
Servings: 4

Ingredients:
- 6 cups beef stock, all organic, store-bought, unsalted
- 2 large garlic cloves, minced
- 1 large celery rib, strings removed, minced
- 1 large shallot, minced
- 1 small carrot, peeled, diced
- 1 can, 15 oz. button mushrooms, pieces and stems, rinsed well, drained
- 1 Tbsp. olive oil
- ½ head white cabbage, cored, tough stems removed, julienned
- ½ pound lean ground beef
- sea salt and white pepper, to taste

For garnish, all optional
- ⅛ cup fresh chives, minced
- A dash of dried pepper flakes

Directions:
1. Pour oil into Dutch oven set over medium heat. Add in and sauté garlic and onion until limp and aromatic. Add in ground beef; stir-fry until seared brown, breaking up larger clumps as you go.
2. Except for garnishes and cabbage, add in remaining ingredients into Dutch oven. Stir. Bring soup to a boil. Secure lid. Turn down heat to the lowest setting. Simmer for 20 minutes.
3. Add in cabbage. Cook for another 10 minutes, covered. Taste; adjust seasoning, if needed. Turn off heat.
4. Ladle soup into bowls. Garnish with fresh chives and pepper flakes, if using. Cool soup slightly before serving.

90. CHICKEN, MUSHROOM AND VEGETABLE SOUP

Prep time: 15 mins
Cook time: 15 mins
Total time: 30 mins
Servings: 6

Ingredients:
- 6 cups mushroom or vegetable stock, all organic, store-bought, unsalted
- 3 large chicken thigh fillets, deboned, diced into bite-sized pieces, rinsed, drained well
- 2 large garlic cloves, peeled, minced
- 2 large shallots, peeled, minced

- ❖ 1 large carrot, peeled, diced
- ❖ 1 large celery rib, strings removed, minced
- ❖ ½ small red bell pepper, ribbed, deseeded, diced
- ❖ 2 Tbsp. olive oil, divided
- ❖ 1 can 15 oz. button mushrooms, pieces and stems, rinsed, drained
- ❖ 1 can 15 oz. straw mushrooms, halved lengthwise, rinsed, drained
- ❖ sea salt and white pepper, to taste

For garnish, all optional
- ❖ ⅛ cup fresh parsley, minced
- ❖ dash dried pepper flakes

Directions:
1. Pour 1 tablespoon of oil into a non-stick skillet set over medium heat. Fry diced chicken until seared and golden on all sides. Transfer partially cooked meat into a large stockpot.
2. Pour remaining oil into skillet. Add in and sauté celery, garlic, and shallots until limp and aromatic. Transfer contents of skillet into a stockpot, along with remaining ingredients. Set stockpot over high heat. Bring soup to a boil. Secure lid.
3. Turn down heat to medium setting; simmer soup for 35 minutes, or until chicken is fork-tender. Turn off heat. Stir. Taste; adjust seasoning, if needed.
4. Ladle soup into individual bowls. Garnish with parsley and pepper flakes, if using. Cool slightly before serving.

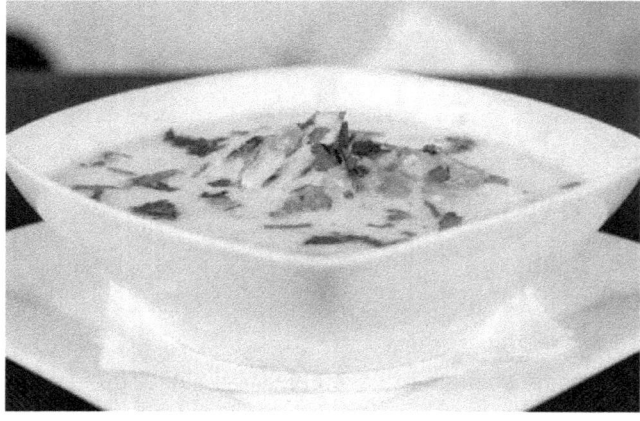

91. Creamy Chicken Curry

Prep Time: 10 mins
Cook Time: 35 mins
Total Time: 45 mins
Serving: 4

Ingredients:
- 4 large chicken thigh fillets, halved
- 2 large garlic clove, peeled, minced
- 2 large shallots, peeled, minced
- 1 thumb-sized ginger, peeled, crushed with the flat side of the knife
- 1 small carrot, peeled, cubed
- 1 small red bell pepper, ribbed, deseeded, cubed
- 1 small sweet potato, peeled, cubed
- 1 banana chili, halved lengthwise, deseeded
- 1 bird's eye chili, halved lengthwise, deseeded
- 2 cups chicken or mushroom stock, all organic, store-bought, unsalted
- 2 cans, 15 oz. each, coconut cream, divided
- 1 can, 15 oz., straw mushrooms, rinsed, drained well
- 1 Tbsp. coconut oil
- 1 Tbsp. *garam masala*
- ½ Tbsp. curry powder
- ¼ tsp. Spanish paprika (for a spicier blend, use Indian paprika)

Garnishes (all optional)
- 2 Tbsp., heaping fresh cilantro, minced
- 1 piece, small lime, sliced into wedges, pips removed

Directions:
1. Pour coconut oil into Dutch oven set over medium heat. Add in and sauté garlic, ginger and shallot until limp and aromatic. Add in chicken thigh fillets; cook until seared on all sides.
2. Except for garnishes and 1 can of coconut cream, add in remaining ingredients into Dutch oven. Stir. Secure lid, and cook until chicken is fork-tender, about 30 minutes. Turn off heat.
3. Pour in remaining can of coconut cream. Taste; adjust seasoning, if needed.
4. Ladle equal portions of curry into bowls. Garnish with cilantro, if using. Serve with a lime wedge. Squeeze lime juice over the dish before eating.

92. CHERRY JAM

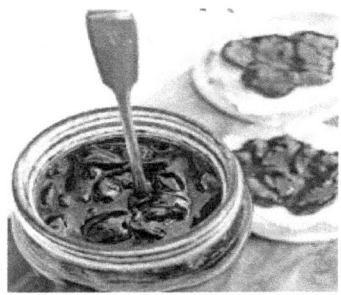

Prep Time: 10 mins
Cook Time: 17 mins
Total Time: 27 mins
Servings: 1

Ingredients:
- 2 lbs tart cherries
- 3 tablespoons balsamic vinegar
- ¼ cup of water
- ½ lemon, freshly squeezed
- 1 cup of raw organic honey

Directions:
1. In a saucepan set over medium heat, combine water, balsamic vinegar, honey, tart cherries, and lemon. Bring to a boil. Reduce heat to a low setting.
2. Using a wooden spoon, mash tart cherries. Stirring frequently until the liquid has evaporated.
3. Turn off the heat. Let cool at room temperature before storing in an airtight jar/container. Use as needed.

93. Apricot Cinnamon Jam

Prep time: 10 mins
Cook time: 45 mins
Total Time: 55 mins
Serves: 1

Ingredients:
- 2 lbs apricots, diced
- 2 tablespoons cinnamon powder
- ½ lemon, freshly squeezed
- 1 cup of raw organic honey
- Pinch of sea salt
- ¼ cup of water

Directions:
1. In a saucepan set over medium heat, combine water, lemon, honey, cinnamon powder, apricots, and salt. Bring to a boil. Reduce heat to a low setting.
2. Using a wooden spoon, mash apricots. Stirring frequently until the liquid has evaporated.
3. Turn off the heat. Let cool at room temperature before storing in an airtight jar/container. Use as needed.

94. Sautéed Apples

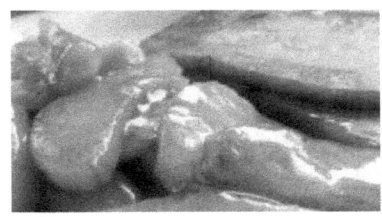

Prep Time: 20 mins
Total Time: 20 mins
Servings: 8

Ingredients:
- 2 tart apples, sliced into wedges
- 1 onion, halved

- ❖ 2 cups dry cider
- ❖ 2 cups vegetable stock
- ❖ Pinch of salt
- ❖ Pinch of pepper

Directions:
1. In a saucepan, combine the onion and cider. Let it boil or until the onions are cooked, and liquid almost is gone.
2. Stir in the apples and stock. Season with salt and pepper. Stir occasionally. Scrape brown bits from the bottom of the pan. Cook for 10 minutes or until the apples are tender and not mushy.

95. PROTEIN CREPES

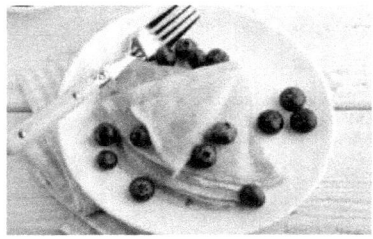

Prep Time: 3 mins
Cook Time: 2mins
Total Time: 5mins
Servings: 1

Ingredients:
- ❖ 2 eggs
- ❖ 2 egg whites
- ❖ ¼ cup coconut flour
- ❖ ½ teaspoon baking soda
- ❖ ¼ cup almond milk
- ❖ 2 tablespoons ground flaxseed

Directions:
1. Heat a large non-stick pan on medium-high. Use cooking spray to coat.
2. Meanwhile, in a food processor, mix all ingredients together. Pour batter into the pan. Swirl it around to make a thin circle.
3. Allow the crepe to cook. Flip crepe over to the other side and cook until both sides are golden brown.

4. Transfer crepe onto a plate and fill with your favourite toppings such as fruits. Fold it and top with more toppings before serving.

96. BANANA CINNAMON SANDWICH

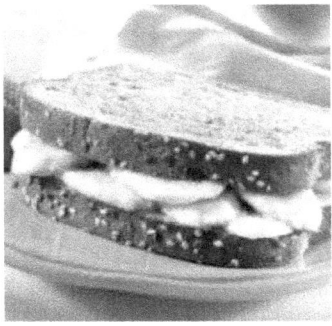

Prep Time: 10 mins
Cook Time: 5 mins
Total Time: 15 mins
Servings: 2

Ingredients:
- 2 rye bread
- Dash of cinnamon powder
- 1 ripe banana, sliced into thin disks

Directions:
1. Place all the banana slices on top of a rye bread slice. Make sure that the bananas are stacked evenly.
2. Sprinkle the cinnamon powder on top of the stacked banana slices. Top with the other slice of rye bread.
3. Place the whole lot in a pre-heated sandwich maker and press down until the bread is toasted. This should take no more than a few seconds.
4. Carefully transfer the sandwich on a plate, and slice in half diagonally. Serve immediately.

97. APPLE PARFAIT

Prep Time: 5mins
Cook Time: 10mins

Total Time: 15mins
Servings: 4

Ingredients:
- 1 tablespoon cashew nuts, chopped

For the Apple jam
- ¾ cup apple juice, unsweetened
- 2 Fuji apples, diced
- 2 tablespoons chia seeds
- ⅛ teaspoon nutmeg powder
- ¾ teaspoon cinnamon powder
- Pinch of sea salt

For the Parfait Base
- 1¼ cups almond milk
- 1 banana, mashed
- ⅛ teaspoon nutmeg powder
- ½ teaspoon cinnamon powder
- 2 tablespoons chia seeds

Directions:
1. In a bowl, combine almond milk, banana, nutmeg powder, cinnamon powder, and chia seeds. Mix until well combined. Chill in the fridge.
2. Meanwhile, in a saucepan set over medium heat. Combine apple juice, apples, nutmeg powder, cinnamon powder, and salt. Bring to a boil. Allow simmering for 20 minutes.
3. Turn off the heat. Mash half of the jam using a wooden spoon. Let cool. Set aside.
4. Spoon 2 tablespoons of parfait base and apple jam into parfait glasses. Garnish with cashew nuts. Serve.

98. OLIVE CROSTINI

Prep Time: 10 mins
Cook Time: 5 mins
Total Time: 15 mins
Servings: 12

Ingredients:
- 2 slices wheat bread, toasted
- 2 garlic cloves, peeled
- 1/8 teaspoon extra virgin olive oil

For the Vegetable Spread
- 1 teaspoon apple cider vinegar
- 1 large black olive in oil, thinly sliced
- 1 roasted red pepper in oil, julienned
- 1 green olive in brine, thinly sliced
- 1/8 cup onion, minced
- 1/4 cup cucumber, julienned
- Pinch of sea salt
- Pinch of black pepper

Directions:
1. Preheat the oven toaster. Rub garlic cloves on the toasted bread. Set aside.
2. In a bowl, combine apple cider vinegar, olive in oil, red pepper in oil, olive in brine, onion, cucumber, salt, and pepper. Adjust seasoning.
3. Spread on bread slices. Place in the oven toaster to warm through. Drizzle in olive oil. Serve.

99. BANANA CINNAMON

Prep time: 2 mins
Cook time: 8 mins
Total time: 10 mins
Servings: 2-4

Ingredients:
- 1 large banana, chopped into 1/2 inch
- 2 tsp. honey
- 1 tsp. cinnamon

Directions:
1. In a small bowl, combine honey and cinnamon.
2. Heat the olive oil in a pan. Cook banana slices for 2 minutes or until browned all over.

3. Pour honey and cinnamon mixture over the bananas. Serve.

100. BANANA CINNAMON COOKIES

Prep Time: 5mins
Cook Time: 10mins
Total Time: 15mins
Servings: 2

Ingredients:
- 2 ripe bananas, peeled
- 2/3 cup applesauce, unsweetened
- ¼ cup almond milk, unsweetened
- 4 pitted dates
- 1 tablespoon cinnamon
- 2/3 cup coconut flour
- 1 teaspoon vanilla
- 1 1/2 teaspoon lemon juice
- 3 tablespoons dried and chopped cranberries
- 1 teaspoon baking powder
- 2 tablespoons dried and chopped raisins

Directions:
1. Preheat the oven to 350 degrees F.
2. In a food processor, combine almond milk, applesauce, dates, and bananas. Blend until you achieve a smooth consistency.
3. Add in coconut flour, baking powder, cinnamon, vanilla, and lemon juice. Blend for 1 minute. Fold in cranberries and raisins.
4. Pour a baking sheet with the cookie dough. Place inside the oven for 20 minutes.
5. Allow to sit for 5 minutes and let it harden. Serve.

101. AVOCADO CHIA PARFAIT

Prep time: 25 mins
Total time: 25 mins
Serves: 2

Ingredients:
- 1 tablespoon cashew nuts, chopped

For the Avocado Jam
- 2 avocados, diced
- 2 tablespoons chia seeds
- ⅛ teaspoon nutmeg powder
- ¾ teaspoon cinnamon powder
- Pinch of sea salt

For the Parfait Base
- 1¼ cups almond milk
- 1 banana, mashed
- ⅛ teaspoon nutmeg powder
- ½ teaspoon cinnamon powder
- 2 tablespoons pumpkin seeds

Directions:
1. In a bowl, combine almond milk, banana, nutmeg powder, cinnamon powder, and pumpkin seeds. Mix until well combined. Chill in the fridge.
2. Meanwhile, in a saucepan set over medium heat. Combine avocados, nutmeg powder, cinnamon powder, and salt. Bring to a boil. Allow simmering for 20 minutes.
3. Turn off the heat. Mash half of the jam using a wooden spoon. Let cool. Set aside.
4. Spoon 2 tablespoons of parfait base and apple jam into parfait glasses. Garnish with cashew nuts. Serve.

102. HONEYED SWEET POTATOES

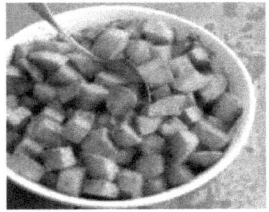

Prep Time: 10 mins.
Cook Timed: 45 mins
Total Time: 55 mins
Servings: 6

Ingredients:
- coconut butter
- 2 large sweet potatoes, sliced into thick cubes
- 2 tablespoons raw organic honey
- ½ cup pecans, toasted
- Pinch of sea salt

Directions:
1. Preheat electric grill.
2. Grease sweet potatoes slivers with coconut butter.
3. Grill until brown on both sides. Remove from heat. Drizzle in honey, pecans, and salt.

103. BANANA DARK ALMONDSCHOCO

Prep Time: 10 mins
Cook Time: 35 mins
Total Time: 45 mins
Servings: 6

Ingredients:
- ½ cup dark chocolate
- 2 bananas, chopped into bite-sized pieces
- Raw almonds, crushed

Directions:
1. Melt the chocolate in a microwave-safe bowl for 1 minute and 30 seconds.
2. Roll chopped bananas on the melted chocolate. Rollover almonds.
3. Refrigerate for 1 hour. Serve.

104. Chocolate Avocado Pudding

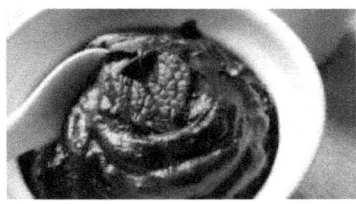

Prep Time 5 mins
Total Time 5 mins
Serving: 4

Ingredients:
- 1 ½ avocado
- 2 tbsp. chia seeds
- 1 cup almond milk, unsweetened
- 2 tbsp. cocoa powder
- 1 pack whey protein powder
- 4 scoops stevia
- Pinch of salt

Directions:
1. Combine avocadoes, chia seeds, almond milk, cocoa powder, whey protein powder, stevia, and salt in a blender. Blend for 2 minutes or until all ingredients are well-combined
2. Refrigerate for 1 hour. Serve.

105. Blueberry Pudding

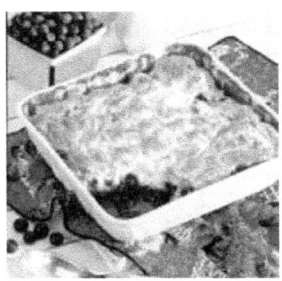

Prep Time: 15 mins.
Cook Time: 45 mins.

Total Time: 1 hr
Servings: 4

Ingredients:
- 3 eggs
- Nonstick cooking spray
- 2 tablespoons maple syrup
- 1 cup blueberry
- 2 teaspoons lemon peel, shredded
- ¼ cup all-purpose flour
- ¼ teaspoon salt
- 3 tablespoons lemon juice
- 1 cup fat-free milk
- 3 tablespoons vegetable spread

Directions:
1. Coat slow cooker with cooking spray. Place the berries and pour maple syrup.
2. Meanwhile, in a bowl, combine maple syrup, lemon peel, flour, and salt. Add lemon juice, milk, and vegetable oil spread. Mix using an electric mixer until well combined. Set aside.
3. In another bowl. Whisk egg whites until soft peaks form. Pour batter over the berries.
4. Cover and cook on high for 2 hours. Cool, uncovered for 1 hour. Serve.

106. APPLE CHIPS

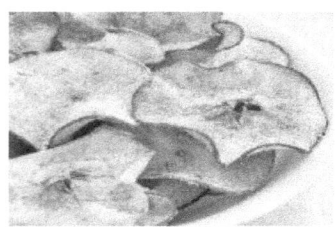

Prep Time: 5 mins
Cook Time: 2 hrs 55 mins
Total Time: 3 hrs
Servings: 2

Ingredients:
- 2 apples, cored, thinly sliced
- Dash of cinnamon

Directions:
1. Preheat the oven to 275 degrees F. Line a cookie sheet with parchment paper.
2. Layer sliced apples in the cookie sheet. Dust with cinnamon.
3. Place inside the oven and bake for 2 hours. Do not forget to flip apple slices every hour.
4. Remove apple chips and let cool. Serve as needed. Leftovers can be stored in an air-tight container.

107. BAKED CINNAMON APPLES

Prep Time 10 mins
Cook Time 1 hr
Total Time 1 hr 10 mins
Servings: 6

Ingredients:
- 4 apples, cored
- ¼ cup raisins
- ½ cup 100% apple juice
- 1/8 tsp. nutmeg
- 1 tbsp. lemon juice
- ½ tsp. ground cinnamon
- 2 tbsp. brown sugar
- 1 tsp. lemon peel, grated

Directions:
1. Layer apples in a baking dish. Fill them with raisins.
2. Meanwhile, in a small bowl, put together apple juice, nutmeg, lemon juice, ground cinnamon, brown sugar, and lemon peel. Mix ingredients until well-combined.
3. Coat apples with the mixture. Cover with plastic wrap. Set aside.
4. For the remaining cinnamon, place inside the microwave and heat for 4 minutes or until the sauce thickens.
5. Drizzle over apples. Serve.

108. Tapenade Crostini

Prep Time: 15 mins
Total Time: 15 mins
Servings: 24

Ingredients:
- 2 slices wheat bread, toasted
- 2 garlic cloves, peeled
- ½ teaspoon extra virgin olive oil

For the Tapenade
- 6 black olives in oil, pitted, minced
- 2 tablespoon golden raisins, soaked in water for 20 minutes
- 1 tablespoon capers in brine, minced
- 1 tablespoon fresh parsley, minced
- 1 tablespoon lime juice, freshly squeezed
- ¼ tablespoon thyme, minced
- Pinch of sea salt
- Pinch of white pepper

Directions:
1. Preheat the oven toaster. Rub garlic cloves on the toasted bread. Set aside.
2. In a small bowl, combine chicken, onion, avocado, celery rib, cashew nuts, salt and pepper. Adjust seasoning.
3. Spread on bread slices. Place in the oven toaster to warm through. Garnish with chives. Serve.

109. Honey Baked Apricots

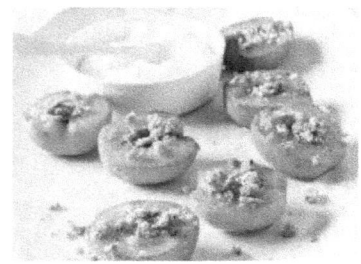

Prep Time: 10 mins

Cook Time: 30 mins
Total Time: 40 mins
Servings: 4

Ingredients:
- olive oil for greasing
- 4 fresh apricots, halved, pitted
- ½ cup walnuts, roughly chopped
- Pinch of sea salt
- ½ cup honey

Directions:
1. Preheat the oven to 350°F.
2. Line a baking dish with parchment paper and grease with oil.
3. Layer apricots and sprinkle walnuts. Season with salt. Season with salt
4. Drizzle honey. Bake for 25 minutes. Remove from heat. Place fruits into individual bowls with nuts.

110. CROSTINI WITH TOMATO SPREAD

Prep Time: 5 mins
Cook Time: 2 hrs 45 mins
Total Time: 2 hrs 50 mins
Servings: 4

Ingredients:
- 2 slices wheat bread, toasted
- 2 garlic cloves, peeled
- ⅛ teaspoon extra virgin olive oil

For the Tomato Spread
- 2 teaspoons lemon juice, freshly squeezed
- 1 fresh oregano leaf, julienned
- 1 green tomato, minced
- 1 red tomato, minced
- Pinch of sea salt
- Pinch of white pepper
- Cayenne powder, optional

Directions:
1. Preheat the oven toaster. Rub garlic cloves on the toasted bread. Set aside.
2. In a small bowl, combine chicken, onion, avocado, celery rib, cashew nuts, salt and pepper. Adjust seasoning.
3. Spread on bread slices. Place in the oven toaster to warm through. Garnish with chives. Serve.

111. SWEET POTATOES IN CREAMY COCONUT SAUCE

Prep time: 10 mins
Cook time: 20 mins
Total Time: 30 mins
Servings: 4

Ingredients:
- coconut butter
- 2 large sweet potatoes, sliced into thick cubes
- 1 can coconut cream
- 1 tablespoon of raw organic honey
- 1 cup fresh blueberries

Directions:
1. Preheat electric grill.
2. Meanwhile, combine coconut cream and honey. Bring to a boil. Stir continuously.
3. Grease sweet potatoes with coconut butter. Grill until brown on both sides. Remove from heat. Drizzle in coconut sauce. Garnish with blueberries. Serve.

112. HONEY BAKED APPLES WITH WALNUTS

Prep Time: 15 mins
Cook Time: 40 mins
Total Time: 55 mins
Servings: 4

Ingredients:
- olive oil for greasing
- 4 small apples, halved
- ½ cup walnuts, roughly chopped
- Pinch of sea salt
- ½ cup honey

Directions:
1. Preheat the oven to 350°F.
2. Line a baking dish with parchment paper and grease with oil.
3. Layer apples and sprinkle walnuts. Season with salt. Season with salt
4. Drizzle honey. Bake for 25 minutes. Remove from heat. Place fruits into individual bowls with nuts.

113. Dark Chocó Almond Butter

Prep Time: 5 mins
Cook Time: 5 mins
Total Time: 10 mins
Serving: 4

Ingredients:
- ½ tsp. baking soda
- 1 cup almond butter
- 1 egg, large
- ¾ cup sugar
- ½ tsp. salt
- ½ cup dark chocolate, chopped

Directions:
1. Preheat the oven to 350 degrees F. Line a baking sheet.
2. Meanwhile, put together baking soda, almond butter, egg, sugar, and salt. Mix until all ingredients are well-combined.
3. Fold in chocolate. Mix until it forms a dough.
4. Spoon an equal amount of mixture on a baking sheet. Place inside the oven and bake for 10 minutes.
5. Allow cookies to cool before serving.

114. Sweet Potato and Chia Butter

Prep Time: 5 mins
Cook Time: 45 mins
Total Time: 50 mins
Serves 2

Ingredients:
- 1 cup of coconut milk
- 1 tablespoon coconut oil, melted
- 1 can, sweet potato puree
- 3 tablespoons raw organic honey
- 1 cup raw pecans, soaked in water overnight
- 2 tablespoon chia seeds
- 2 vanilla pods, halved lengthwise
- 1½ teaspoon cinnamon powder
- ½ teaspoon ginger powder
- ¼ teaspoon nutmeg powder
- Pinch of salt

Directions:
1. Place coconut milk, coconut oil, sweet potato puree, honey, pecans, chia seeds, vanilla pods, cinnamon powder, ginger powder, nutmeg, and salt into a food processor.
2. Process until smooth. Transfer into an airtight container. Use as needed.

115. Chia Bread

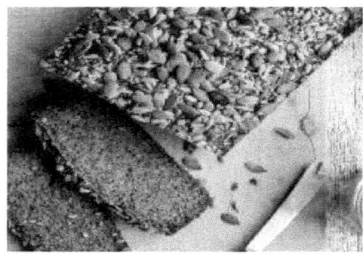

Prep Time 20 mins

Cook Time 45 mins
Total Time 1 hr 5 mins
Servings: 6

Ingredients:

- coconut oil for greasing
- 3 cups almond flour
- 1½ teaspoon baking soda
- ⅓ cup arrowroot powder
- ½ tablespoon chia seed, coarsely ground
- ½ teaspoon of sea salt
- ¾ cup coconut cream
- 5 eggs, whisked
- 1½ teaspoons coconut vinegar
- ½ cup butter, melted
- 1 teaspoon chia seeds, whole

Directions:

1. Preheat oven to 350°F.
2. Lightly grease loaf tin with coconut oil.
3. Combine almond flour, baking soda, arrowroot powder, ground chia seeds, and salt in a bowl. Make a well in the centre. Pour coconut cream, eggs, vinegar, and butter. Stir until well combined. Pour into a loaf tin. Sprinkle whole chia seeds on top.
4. Bake for 30 minutes or until a toothpick inserted in centre comes out clean. Remove from the oven and let cool. Serve.

116. CROSTINI ARUGULA AND SPINACH

Prep Time: 15 mins
Cook Time: 30 mins
Total Time: 45 mins
Servings: 20

Ingredients:

- 2 slices wheat bread, toasted
- 2 garlic cloves, peeled

For the Toppings:
- 2 tablespoons water
- 1 teaspoon Dijon mustard
- 1 teaspoon apple cider vinegar
- 1 handful babyspinach leaves
- 1 handful arugula leaves
- Pinch of sea salt
- Pinch of white pepper

Directions:
1. Rub garlic cloves on the toasted bread. Set aside.
2. Whisk Dijon mustard and apple cider vinegar. Stir until the dressing blends and emulsifies. Tip in spinach and arugula leaves. Season with salt and pepper. Serve.

117. PEPPER PIZZA

Prep Time: 10mins
Cook Time: 20 mins
Total Time: hrs 30 min
Servings: 4

Ingredients:
- 1 slice pizza loaf, toasted
- 1 tablespoon Basil-Tomato Pesto Sauce
- ½ tablespoon red bell pepper, julienned
- ½ tablespoon onion, julienned
- ½ cup baby spinach
- 1 teaspoon extra virgin oil
- 1 tablespoon Cashew Cheese
- Pinch of salt
- Pinch of black pepper

Directions:
1. Spread basil-tomato pesto sauce on one side of the bread. Layer onions and baby spinach on top.

2. Drizzle olive oil and sprinkle cashew cheese. Season with salt and black pepper. Heat in a toaster oven. Serve.

118. Grilled Plantains

Prep Time: 5 mins
Cook Time: 30 mins
Total Time: 35 mins
Servings: 4

Ingredients:
- ¼ cup coconut flakes, toasted
- 4 ripe plantains, peeled, quartered lengthwise
- ¼ cup almond flakes, toasted
- Coconut butter, for greasing

Directions:
1. Preheat electric grill.
2. Grease plantain slivers with coconut butter.
3. Grill until brown on both sides. Remove from heat. Drizzle in coconut flakes and almond.

119. Sweet Potato Matchsticks

Prep Time: 15 mins
Cook Time: 15 mins
Total Time: 35 mins
Servings: 4

Ingredients:
- 2 sweet potatoes, sliced into thick matchsticks
- 1 tablespoon of raw organic honey
- ½ cup fresh blackberries
- coconut butter
- ¼ cup cashew nuts, chopped

Directions:
1. Preheat electric grill.
2. Grease sweet potatoes slivers with coconut butter.
3. Grill until brown on both sides. Remove from heat. Drizzle in honey, blueberries, and cashew nuts.

120. CAULIFLOWER POPPERS

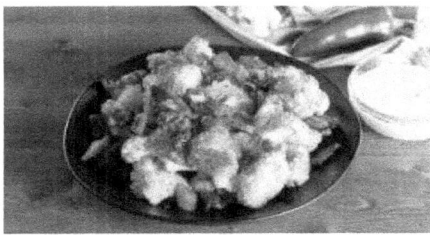

Prep Time: 10 mins
Cook Time: 35 mins
Total Time: 45 mins
Servings: 6

Ingredients:
- 2 cauliflower heads, sliced into bite-sized florets
- Dash of paprika
- Pinch of sea salt
- olive oil, for drizzling

Directions:
1. Preheat the oven to 425°F.
2. Line 1 baking sheet with aluminium foil.
3. Layer cauliflower on baking sheets. Drizzle in oil. Season with paprika and sea salt.
4. Bake for 1 hour. Flip veggies every now and then. Let cool. Serve.

121. Breaded Blossoms

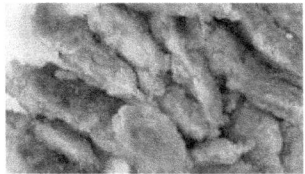

Prep Time: 25 mins
Cook Time: 20 mins
Total Time: 45 mins
Servings: 4

Ingredients:
- 2 lbs zucchini blossoms
- balsamic vinegar, for drizzling
- 1 cup almond flour
- olive oil
- Pinch of sea salt

Directions:
1. In a skillet set over medium heat, pour oil. Swirl pan to coat. Season zucchini blossoms with salt. Dredge in almond flour.
2. Cook breaded blossoms until crisp and golden. Drain on paper towels. Drizzling balsamic vinegar. Serve.

122. Crostini Garlic

Prep Time: 10 mins
Cook Time: 20 mins
Total Time::30mins
Servings: 10

Ingredients:
- 4 garlic cloves, peeled
- 4 slices wheat bread, toasted
- ⅛ teaspoon extra virgin olive oil

For the Vegetable Spread
- ❖ 1 teaspoon apple cider vinegar
- ❖ Pinch of black pepper
- ❖ 1 red pepper in oil, roasted, julienned
- ❖ 1 green olive in brine, sliced thinly
- ❖ 2 black olives in oil, sliced thinly
- ❖ ⅛ cup onion, minced
- ❖ ¼ cup cucumber, julienned
- ❖ Pinch of sea salt

Directions:
1. Preheat the oven toaster. Rub garlic cloves on the toasted bread. Set aside.
2. In a bowl, combine apple cider vinegar, olive in oil, red pepper in oil, olive in brine, onion, cucumber, salt, and pepper. Adjust seasoning.
3. Spread on bread slices. Place in the oven toaster to warm through. Drizzle in olive oil. Serve.

---

123. CHICKEN ENCHILADAS

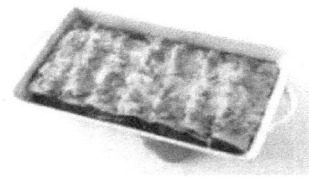

Prep Time: 1 hr
Cook Time: 15 mins
Total Time: 1 hr 15 mins
Servings: 3

Ingredients:

For the Chicken
- ❖ 1 lb. chicken breasts
- ❖ 1 garlic clove, chopped
- ❖ 1/4 yellow onion, chopped finely
- ❖ 2 tbsp. olive oil
- ❖ Pinch of sea salt

For the Sauce
- ❖ 3 garlic cloves, chopped
- ❖ 1 1/2 lbs. tomatillos, husks removed
- ❖ 1 Poblano pepper
- ❖ 1 Serrano chili
- ❖ 1/8 cup cooking fat
- ❖ Pinch of sea salt

For the Enchiladas
- ❖ 8 tortillas
- ❖ 1/2 cup sour cream, preferably made in cashew
- ❖ 1 cup raw cheese, shredded
- ❖ 1/2 cup Queso Fresco, crumbled

Directions:
1. For the chicken, place 2 tablespoons cooking oil in a deep frying pan and sauté garlic and onions. Continue sautéing until brown. Measure a teaspoon of salt and season chicken breasts.
2. Place them on heated oil and fry. Cook until both sides are brown in colour. Set aside.
3. For the sauce, combine chiles and tomatillos in a saucepan. Pour water until the first ingredients are completely covered by water.
4. Set stove in medium-high heat and bring to a boil. Continue boiling for 15 minutes.
5. Get the Poblano chili and roast in a broiler. Turn to roast each side evenly. Take out of the oven and put inside a plastic bag. Store for 15 minutes. It will produce steam that will help skin removal easily.
6. Take the chili out of the bag then peel. Cut in half then scrape off seeds. Place the remaining chili in a food processor. Strain tomatillos and chilies.
7. Add to processor together with garlic. Process until it forms a smooth, saucy texture.
8. Heat oil in a saucepan. Once it's smoking, add tomatillo sauce. Stir constantly until it simmers and forms small bubbles. Decrease heat and continue simmering for five minutes until the sauce thickens. Add a tablespoon of sea salt.
9. Get the pre-cooked chicken and drop them into the sauce. Continue simmering for 45 minutes until it completely cooks. Scoop out chicken and shred.
10. Measure a cup of sauce for later use. Bring the chicken back and season according to preference. Continue simmering while assembling the meal.
11. For the enchiladas, preheat oven (350 degrees Fahrenheit). Put a spoonful of chicken-sauce mixture on the tortilla then top with a dash of cheese. Roll up and flip.

12. Grease a casserole dish then place the tortilla rolls in it. Pack them together tightly to keep them from unravelling. Broken tortillas and excess sauces can be placed on the sides to fill the spaces in the casserole. Pour reserved sauce on the tortillas then top with cheese.
13. Bake for 15 minutes until the cheese melts. Top with cream, sprinkle with Queso Fresco and serve hot.

124. CASHEW BUTTER

Prep Time: 10 mins
Cook Time: 15 mins
Total Time: 25 mins
Servings: 2

Ingredients:
- 1½ cups raw cashew nuts halved
- ½ cup coconut flakes, unsweetened
- 2 tablespoons sesame seeds
- 1 tablespoon coconut oil
- ¼ teaspoon of sea salt

Directions:
1. Preheat the oven to 350°F.
2. Line a baking sheet with aluminum foil. Spread sesame seeds nuts, coconut flakes, and cashew nuts on the baking sheet. Bake for 10 minutes or until golden brown.
3. Remove from heat. Cool before placing into a food processor. Pour olive oil and salt. Process until smooth. Store in an airtight container.

125. BURRITOS

Prep Time: 15 mins
Cook Time: 30 mins
Total Time: 45
Servings: 4

Ingredients:

Chili Beef
- 2 cups lean ground beef
- 1 white onion, diced
- 3 garlic cloves, diced
- 1 can tomato passata
- 1 tsp. coriander seeds powder
- 1 long red chili, diced
- 2 tsp. cumin powder
- 1 1/2 tsp. sweet paprika
- Pinch of sea salt
- 1 tbsp. olive oil

Salsa Salad
- 2 tomatoes, quartered
- 1 garlic clove, minced
- 1/2 cup spring onion, diced
- 1 cucumber, diced
- 1 red chili, chopped
- Avocado, cut into quarters
- 2/3 cups red peppers, diced
- 1/2 cup coriander, chopped
- Olive oil
- Pinch of sea salt

Sweet Potato
- 2 sweet potatoes, cubed
- 1/2 tsp. cumin powder
- 1 tsp. smoked paprika
- Olive oil
- Pinch of salt
- Pinch of pepper

Directions:
1. Preheat oven (390 degrees Fahrenheit). Get a casserole dish or large deep pan and place over medium heat. Heat a tablespoon of cooking fat and sauté onions until golden brown and soft.
2. Increase heat to high and add beef in small batches then break it into ground pieces. Stir and cook for 5 to 7 minutes until brown. Add the spices in the beef ingredients, chili, garlic and season with salt. Let the mixture cook for several more minutes.
3. Add tomato passata. You can also use canned diced tomatoes of the same amount with water drained. Pour half-cup of water. Stir to mix ingredients and bring to a boil.

4. Reduce heat to low medium and simmer for 25 minutes while stirring occasionally.
5. Prepare the roasted sweet potatoes by combining sweet potatoes, cumin, sweet paprika and 2 tbsps. Olive oil. Toss until sweet potatoes are completely coated. Spread in a baking tray.
6. Bake in 190 C d f oven heat for 15 minutes. Remove from the oven and season with the desired amount of salt and pepper. Toss to coat sweet potatoes evenly. Place back to the oven and bake for another 5 minutes
7. Prepare the salad while the rest of the ingredients are cooking. Combine tomatoes, red peppers, and cucumbers in a salad bowl. Add garlic, coriander, spring onion, and chopped chili. Season with salt, limejuice and two tablespoons olive oil. Toss together until ingredients are mixed completely. Set aside.
8. Get an avocado as an additional ingredient or garnishing. Cut it into four quarters and drizzle with a small amount of limejuice. This will keep avocados from discoloring. Divide all ingredient mixes into four serving bowls and place one-quarter of avocado each. Garnish with a slice of lime, if preferred.

126. TOFU PATTIES

Prep: 15 mins
Cook: 10 mins
Total Time: 25 mins
Servings: 8

Ingredients:
- 14 oz. tofu extra, firm
- 1 onion, diced
- 1 teaspoon garlic powder
- 2 tablespoons spelt flour
- 1 tablespoon soy sauce
- 2 green onions, diced
- Pinch of ground black pepper

Directions:
1. Crumble tofu in a bowl, and then mix in the remaining ingredients.
2. Season with black pepper then mixes well. Refrigerate for at least half an hour.
3. Preheat grill pan over medium flame. Coat with coconut oil.

CHAPTER 5 - ANTI-INFLAMMATORY: RARE SLOW COOKED MEALS

127. BEEF BORSCHT

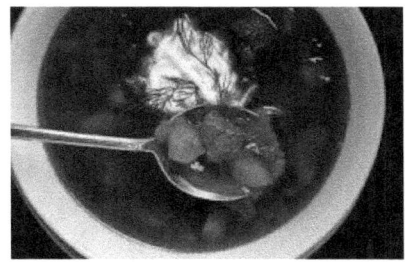

Prep Time: 20 mins
Cook Time: 4 hrs. 30 mins
Total Time: 4 hrs. 50 mins
Servings: 8

Ingredients:

- 2 cups beef bone broth
- ½ pound beef shank, quartered
- 1 piece, large red beets, peeled, cubed
- 1 piece, carrot, cubed
- 1 can dice and peeled tomatoes
- ¼ tsp. tomato paste
- ¼ tsp. garlic powder
- 1 piece, medium onion, minced
- Pinch of sugar
- Pinch of sea salt
- Pinch of black pepper, to taste
- ½ piece, small cabbage, cored, leaves julienned

Directions:

1. Pour beef bone broth, beef shank, large red beets, carrots, tomatoes, tomato paste, garlic powder, onion, and sugar. Season with salt and pepper.
2. Secure the lid. Cook on high for 4 hours. Adjust taste if needed.
3. Before the end of cooking time, tip in the cabbage. Secure the lid and cook for another 30 minutes.
4. Serve by ladling into soup bowls.

128. PORK AND BEEF SPICE

Prep Time 5 mins
Total Time 5 mins
Servings: 6

Ingredients:
- 2 tablespoons olive oil
- 2 garlic cloves, minced
- 1 onion, minced
- ½ pound streaky bacon, diced
- 1 pound ground beef
- 1 pound ground pork
- 1 cup beef bone broth
- 1 can peel and diced tomatoes
- 2 fresh jalapeño pepper, minced
- 1 tablespoon dried oregano, crumbled
- 2 tablespoons chili powder
- 1 fresh bird's eye chili, minced
- 1 tablespoon cayenne powder
- Dash of red pepper flakes
- ⅛ tablespoon black pepper
- 8 oz. natural cheddar cheese curd
- Pinch of sea salt, only if needed

Directions:
1. Heat the oil in a skillet. Sauté garlic and onion for 3 minutes. Cook bacon for 3 minutes or until crisp. Tip in ground beef and pork. Stir in ground pork and beef. Cook for four minutes or until both is,

brown all over. Transfer contents of the skillet into the crockpot slow cooker.
2. Pour beef broth, tomatoes, beef broth, jalapeño pepper, dried oregano, chili powder, bird's eye chili, cayenne powder, red pepper flakes, and black pepper. Secure the lid. Cook on low for 8 hours.
3. Turn off the heat. Add cheese curds. Adjust seasoning if needed. Ladle into bowls. Serve.

129. CREAMY PORK STEW IN YOGURT SAUCE

Prep Time 15 mins
Cook Time: 2hr
Total Time 2 hrs. 15 mins
Servings: 8

Ingredients:

- 1 ½ lb. lean pork, sliced into chunks
- 3 garlic cloves, crushed
- 1 large onion, chopped
- 1 ½ tsp dried turmeric
- 1 ½ tsp dried coriander
- ¾ tsp dried oregano
- ¾ tsp freshly ground black pepper
- 21 oz. chopped tomatoes
- 1 ½ Tbsp. pureed tomato
- 21 oz. canned chickpeas, drained thoroughly
- Pinch of sea salt
- 21 oz. fresh spinach, chopped
- 1 tbsp. lemon zest, freshly grated
- 3 tbsp. low-fat Greek yoghurt

Directions:

1. Heat oil in a nonstick skillet. Once hot, add pork. Cook for 5 minutes or until brown on all sides. Transfer cooked pork into a platter lined with paper towels.
2. In the same skillet, sauté onion for 2 minutes or until translucent. Transfer into the crockpot slow cooker.

3. Meanwhile, in a medium-sized mixing bowl, combine dried oregano, coriander, turmeric, and black pepper. Add tomatoes, garlic, pureed tomatoes, and chickpeas. Mix well. Season with salt.
4. Put the pork into the crockpot slow cooker and pour the mixture. Secure the lid. Cover and cook on low for 6 hours.
5. 30 minutes before the 6th-hour mark, put lemon zest and spinach. Cover the lid and cook on high for 30 minutes. Transfer to a serving dish. Put a dollop of yoghurt. Serve.

130. RUM PORK SHOULDER

Prep Time 5 mins
Total Time 5 mins
Servings: 4

Ingredients:

- 3 lbs. boneless pork shoulder, trimmed
- 5 garlic cloves, cut into thin slivers
- 2 gingerroot, cut into thin slivers
- 1 tsp. dry mustard
- 2 tbsp. coconut sugar
- 1 lime juice, zested, freshly squeezed
- ½ cup dry rum
- 1 tsp. sea salt
- 1 tsp. cracked black peppercorns
- ½ chili pepper, minced
- 1 tbsp. arrowroot, dissolved in 2 tablespoons cold water

Directions:

1. Prepare pork shoulder by making small slits on the sides of the meat. Insert garlic and ginger slivers into the sides.
2. Make small slits on all sides of the meat, insert ginger and garlic slivers.
3. Meanwhile, prepare a mixing bowl. Mix coconut sugar and mustard. Rub mixture all over the pork shoulder. Transfer pork into the broiler and broil for 15 minutes.
4. Next, transfer broiled pork into the slow cooker. Secure the lid. Cook on low for 6 hours.

5. In another bowl, mix rum, limejuice, salt, and pepper. Before the 6th hour mark, pour the mixture into the pork. Secure the lid. Cook on high for another 1 hour.
6. Remove from the crockpot and add arrowroot mixture and chili pepper. Serve with the slow-cooked pork.

131. Braised Pork Shanks

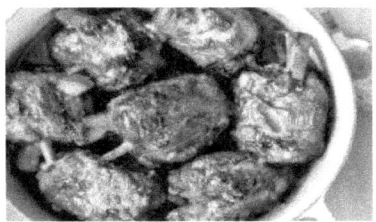

Prep Time: 1 hr.
Cook Time: 2 hr. 30 mins
Total Time: 3 hr. 30 mins
Servings: 6

Ingredients:
- 2 tablespoons olive oil
- 4 large pork shanks, patted dry
- 3 onions, finely chopped
- 6 garlic cloves, minced
- 2 carrots, diced
- 2 stalks celery, diced
- 1 teaspoon dried thyme
- 1 teaspoon of sea salt
- 1 teaspoon cracked black peppercorns
- 1 cup dry white wine
- 1 can tomatoes with juice
- 1 cup pork stock

Directions:
1. Heat the oil in a nonstick skillet set over medium heat. Cook pork shanks for 10 minutes or until all batches have been cooked through and browned all over. Transfer cooked pork into the crockpot slow cooker.
2. Add remaining oil, sauté onion, garlic, carrots, celery, and thyme. Season with salt and pepper. Cook for 4 minutes. Pour wine. Transfer contents of the skillet into the crockpot slow cooker.

3. Add tomatoes with juice and pork stock. Cover the lid and cook on low for 6 hours.
4. Serve with lemon zest and parsley.

132. Stewing Beef with Horseradish Cream

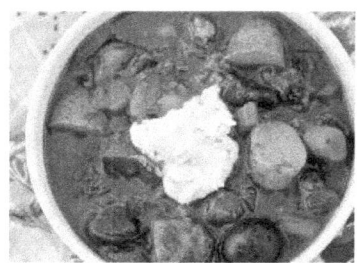

Prep time: 30 mins
Cook Time: 2 hrs.
Total time: 2 hrs. 30 mins
Servings: 6

Ingredients:
- 2 tablespoons olive oil
- 2 lbs. stewing beef, trimmed
- 3 garlic cloves, minced
- 2 onions, finely chopped
- 1 bay leaf
- 2 celery stalks, diced
- ½ teaspoon of sea salt
- ½ teaspoon cracked black peppercorns
- 4 whole cloves
- 8 whole allspice
- 1 cup dry red wine
- 1 tablespoon red wine vinegar
- 3 cups beef stock
- 1 tablespoon coconut sugar
- 4 medium beets, cubed
- 1/2 cup crème Fraiche
- 2 tablespoons homemade horseradish

Directions:

1. Heat the oil in a nonstick skillet set over medium-high heat. Cook the beef for 6 minutes or until browned all over. Transfer cooked beef into the crockpot slow cooker.
2. In the same skillet, sauté garlic and onion. Add bay leaf and celery. Season with salt and pepper.
3. Next, you would need to tie the allspice and garlic cloves using a cheesecloth. Transfer into the slow cooker. Tie cloves and allspice in a cheesecloth. Add to the pan. Pour the wine, vinegar, stock, and coconut sugar. Bring to a boil.
4. Transfer everything into the slow cooker. Stir in beets. Secure the lid. Cook on low for 6 hours.
5. Turn off the heat. Discard bay leaf, allspice, and cloves.
6. Meanwhile, in a bowl, combine crème Fraiche and horseradish. Stir well. Serve with beef.

133. KING PRAWN CURRY

Prep Time: 5 mins
Cook Time: 25 mins
Total Time: 30 mins
Servings: 2

Ingredients:
- 2 lbs. raw king prawns, peeled and deveined
- 2 small onions, chopped
- 5 garlic cloves, crushed
- 12 oz. halved cherry tomatoes
- 1 ½ cups sieved tomatoes
- 12 oz. frozen peas
- 1 ½ tsp sunflower oil
- Pinch of sea salt
- Pinch of ground black pepper
- 3 tbsp. chopped fresh cilantro

Directions:
1. Layer prawns inside the crockpot slow cooker. Spread garlic, onion, cherry tomatoes, sieved tomatoes, and peas all over the prawns. Pour sunflower oil.

2. Secure the lid. Cook on high for 4 hours. Transfer to a serving dish. Sprinkle cilantro. Serve.

134. COD TAGINE

Prep Time: 50 mins
Cook Time: 1 hr.
Total Time: 3hr 50 m
Servings: 8

Ingredients:
- 1 ½ tbsp. paprika
- 1 ½ tsp ground ginger
- 1 ½ tbsp. ground cumin
- 1 cup olive oil
- 1/3 cup dry white wine
- 3 tbsp. fresh cilantro, chopped
- 1/3 cup lemon juice, freshly squeezed
- Pinch of sea salt
- 2 ¼ lb. cod, washed, sliced into equal portions
- 3 large onions, diced
- 5 garlic cloves, minced
- 2/3 cup seafood or vegetable stock
- ¾ cup sliced pimiento-stuffed green olives
- 3 bay leaves
- Cayenne pepper
- Freshly ground black pepper

Directions:
1. In a small mixing bowl, put together ground ginger, paprika, and cumin. Set aside.
2. In another bowl, combine oil, wine, spice mix, cilantro, lemon juice, salt, and cayenne. In a resalable freezer bag, mix ¾ cup of oil with the lemon juice, wine, cilantro, spice mix, and a pinch of salt and

cayenne. Transfer contents in a zip lock bag. Place the cod fillets inside. Marinate and put inside the freezer for 2 hours.
3. Once ready, pour contents of the zip lock bag including the marinade into the slow cooker. Layer onion and garlic.
4. Secure the lid. Cook on low for 6 hours. Turn off the heat. Discard bay leaves. Transfer to a platter. Serve.

135. Lamb Bone Broth

Prep Time: 5 mins
Cook Time: 6 hrs.
Total Time: 6 hours 5 mins
Servings: 6

Ingredients:

- 4 tablespoons olive oil
- 4 lbs. raw lamb bones with marrow
- 4 garlic cloves, crushed
- 2 white onions, peeled, roughly chopped
- 3 carrots, roughly chopped
- 2 celery stalks, chopped
- 4 tablespoons coconut vinegar
- 2 fresh bay leaves, whole
- 1 handful fresh mint, rinsed, spun-dried
- water
- Pinch of sea salt
- Pinch of black pepper

Directions:

1. Pour half the oil in a non-stick skillet. Fry lamb bones until brown on all sides. Place beef into the slow cooker.
2. Pour the remaining oil and sauté garlic and onion until translucent and fragrant. Add in carrots and celery. Cook until lightly seared. Transfer contents into the slow cooker.
3. Pour coconut vinegar and hot water until all ingredients are submerged underwater.
4. Cover with the lid. Cook bone broth for 6 hours. Turn off heat. Add mint leaves. Allow steeping for 15 minutes.

5. Discard solids and strain the broth. Season with salt and pepper. Serve.

136. TURKEY BONE BROTH

Prep Time: 5 mins
Cook Time: 1 day
Total Time: 1 day 5 mins

Ingredients:
- 2 lbs. roasted turkey bones/carcass
- 2 garlic cloves, crushed
- 2 red onions, peeled, chopped
- 2 celery stalks, chopped
- 1 lemon, halved, freshly squeezed, include lemon rinds
- 1 tablespoon whole peppercorns
- 2 dried bay leaves
- 1 pinch fresh rosemary, roughly torn
- 1 pinch fresh thyme, roughly torn
- Water
- Pinch of sea salt
- Pinch of black pepper

Directions:
1. Place turkey bones, garlic, onions, celery, lemon and lemon rinds, whole peppercorns, bay leaves, rosemary, and thyme into the slow cooker.
2. Pour water until all ingredients are submerged underwater secure lid. Cook on low for 6 hours. Turn off heat. Tip in lemon juice.
3. Discard solids and strain the broth. Season with salt and pepper. Serve.

137. ODDS AND ENDS BEEF STEW

Prep Time: 20 mins
Cook Time: 8 hrs.
Total Time: 8 hrs. 20 mins

Ingredients:
- 4 cups beef bone broth
- 1 thumb-sized ginger, crushed
- 2 onions, quartered
- 1 lb. oxtails, trimmed well
- 1 lb. ox tripe, sliced into inch thick squares
- 2 leeks, green parts minced
- 2 lemongrass bulbs, crushed
- 1 tablespoon black peppercorns
- 1 teaspoon fish sauce

Directions:
1. Pour bone broth and add ginger, onions, oxtails, ox tripe, leeks, lemongrass, black peppercorns, and fish sauce into the slow cooker. Cover the lid and cook on low for 6 hours or until the oxtail is tender. Turn off heat.
2. Reposition the lid and cook for another 30 minutes. Allow resting. Taste; adjust seasoning if needed.
3. Ladle soup into bowls. Serve.

138. SWEDISH MEATBALLS

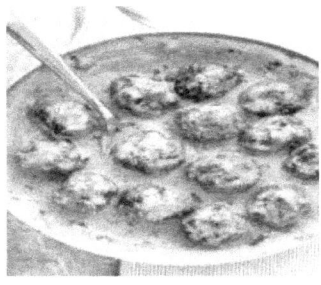

Prep Time: 10 mins
Cook Time: 20 mins

Total Time: 30 mins
Servings: 4

Ingredients:
- 1 lb. lean ground beef
- 1 onion, grated
- 1 egg beaten
- ½ cup almond flour
- 2 teaspoons lemon juice, freshly squeezed
- ½ teaspoon of sea salt
- ½ teaspoon freshly ground black pepper
- ½ teaspoon allspice
- 2 tablespoons extra virgin olive oil
- 1 tablespoon coconut flour
- 1.2 teaspoon cracked black peppercorns
- 2 cups beef stock
- ½ cup sour cream
- 1.2 cup dill funds, chopped

Directions:
1. Combine ground beef, onion, egg, almond flour, lemon juice, zest, salt, pepper, and allspice in a bowl. Mix well. Shape into balls.
2. In a skillet, heat the oil. Cook meatballs in batches for 4 minutes or until browned on all sides. Transfer into the slow cooker. Add coconut flour into the pan and peppercorns. In addition, beef stock. Stir well.
3. Cover the lid and cook on low for 6 hours or on high for 3 hours. Transfer meatballs into a serving dish. Top with sour cream and dill. Serve.

---

139. SAVORY COCOA-FLAVORED BABY BACK RIBS

Prep Time: 10 mins
Cook Time: 3 hrs.
Total Time: 3hrs 10 mins

Ingredients:
- 3 pounds pork baby back ribs

Dry rub
- 2 tablespoons of sea salt
- 2 tablespoons onion powder
- 1 tablespoon garlic powder
- 1 tablespoon ginger powder
- 1 tablespoon cayenne powder
- 2 tablespoons smoky paprika powder
- 1 tablespoon cinnamon powder
- 1 tablespoon oregano powder
- 1 tablespoon mustard powder
- ½ cup unsweetened cocoa powder
- ½ tablespoon white pepper
- ¼ tablespoon red pepper flakes

Directions:
1. Combine sea salt, onion powder, garlic powder, ginger powder, cayenne powder, smoky paprika powder, cinnamon powder, oregano powder, mustard powder, and cocoa powder, white pepper, and red pepper flakes in a bowl. Mix well. Rub generously all over baby back ribs.
2. Place ribs inside the slow cooker. Cover the lid and cook on low for 8 hours. Slice ribs between bones. Serve.

140. TUNA IN BRINE

Prep Time: 5 mins
Cook Time: 15 mins
Total Time: 20 mins

Ingredients:
- 12 oz. canned tuna packed in brine, drained thoroughly
- 3 cups frozen peas
- 12 oz. fresh button mushrooms, sliced thinly
- 3 tbsp. organic butter or ghee
- 1/3 cup rice flour
- 1 ½ cups vegetable or chicken stock
- 1 ½ cups low fat or nut-based milk
- ¾ cup freshly grated Parmesan cheese
- ¾ tsp sea salt

- ❖ ¾ tsp freshly ground black pepper

Directions:
1. Pour tuna in brine into the crockpot slow cooker. Scatter peas and mushrooms.
2. Meanwhile, heat the butter in a saucepan. Once hot and melted, stir in flour. Pour vegetable broth and milk. Mix well. Add in cheese.
3. Once the mixture is hot, pour onto the slow cooker. Season with salt and pepper. Mix well. Secure the lid. Cook on low for 8 hours or on high for 4 hours.
4. Serve with pasta or over a bed of hot rice.

141. SEAFOOD STEW

Prep Time: 1 hr.
Cook Time: 30 mins
Total Time: 1 hr. 30 mins
Servings: 6

Ingredients:
- ❖ ¼ cup olive oil
- ❖ 2 pieces, large garlic clove, minced
- ❖ 1 tsp. dried pepper flakes
- ❖ 1 piece, large   fresh bay leaf
- ❖ 3 cups of fish bone broth
- ❖ ½ cup fresh basil leaves, roughly torn
- ❖ 2½ pounds clams, shells scrubbed clean
- ❖ 1½ pounds green mussels, shells scrubbed clean
- ❖ 1 pound prawns, peeled, deveined, halved lengthwise
- ❖ 1 can, 15 oz. diced and peeled tomatoes
- ❖ ⅛ tsp. fish sauce
- ❖ ½ tsp. white sugar
- ❖ Pinch of sea salt, to taste
- ❖ ⅛ cup fresh parsley, minced, for garnish, optional

Directions:
1. Pour oil into the crockpot slow cooker. Cook garlic, pepper flakes, and bay leaf for 1 minute.

2. Pour fish bone broth, basil leaves, clams, mussels, and prawns. Tip in tomatoes. Season with fish sauce, sugar, and salt.
3. Secure the lid. Cook on high for 4 hours.
4. Discard shells that did not open. Turn off heat.
5. Serve by ladling equal portions into bowls. Garnish with parsley.

142. VEAL ROAST

Prep Time: 10 mins
Cook Time: 2 hrs. 15 mins
Total Time: 2 hrs. 25 mins
Servings: 8

Ingredients:
- 3 tablespoons olive oil, divided
- 2½ pounds veal shoulder, bone-in
- 1 pound fresh porcini mushrooms, sliced into ¼-inch pieces
- ¾ cup of water
- 2 cups beef bone broth
- 3 tablespoons balsamic vinegar
- 1 leek, minced
- ¼ cup red bell pepper, julienned
- Pinch of sea salt
- Pinch of black pepper to taste

Directions:
1. Pour half of the olive oil into the skillet. Cook veal shoulders until brown on all sides. Set aside. Tip in mushrooms and cook until lightly brown on both sides. Transfer into the slow cooker.
2. Pour water, bone broth, balsamic vinegar, leek, red bell pepper, salt, and pepper into the slow cooker. Cover the lid and cook on low for 6 hours.
3. Turn off heat. Transfer meat for carving. Allow sitting for 10 minutes before thinly slicing. Arrange on a platter. Serve.

143. PORK WITH TOMATOES

Total Time: 75 mins
Prep Time: 15 mins
Cook Time: 60 mins
Servings: 6

Ingredients:
- 2 teaspoons olive oil
- 3/4 pound pork tenderloin, fat trimmed, sliced into half-inch round
- ¼ cup shallots, finely chopped
- 14 ½ ounces tomatoes, fire-roasted, crushed
- ½ cup chicken broth
- 3 cups spinach
- 2 tablespoons balsamic vinegar

Directions:
1. Heat oil in a skillet. Cook tenderloin slices for 4 minutes on each side. Transfer into the slow cooker.
2. Stir in shallots, tomatoes, chicken broth, spinach, and balsamic vinegar into the slow cooker. Cover the lid and cook on low for 6 hours.
3. Turn off heat. Adjust taste, if needed. Serve.

144. BALSAMIC PORK

Prep Time: 10 mins
Cook Time: 10 mins
Total Time: 20 mins
Servings: 6

Ingredients:
- 2 teaspoons olive oil
- 4 pork loin chops, five-ounce, boneless, w/ fat trimmed
- ½ teaspoon salt
- 1/3 cup vinegar, balsamic
- 3 twists black pepper, freshly ground
- 1 garlic clove, minced
- ½ cup chicken broth, low-sodium, fat-free

Directions:
1. Pour oil into the skillet. Cook pork loin chops for 4 minutes or until lightly brown on all sides. Transfer into the slow cooker.
2. In the same skillet, sauté garlic for 2 minutes or until fragrant. Transfer into the slow cooker.
3. Pour balsamic vinegar and chicken broth. Cover the lid and cook on low for 4 hours.

4. Turn off heat. Adjust taste, if needed. Serve.

145. BRAISED BRISKET

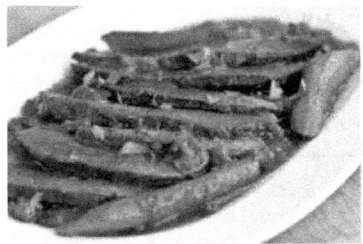

Prep Time: 30 mins
Cook Time: 3 hrs. 30 mins
Total Time: 4 hrs.
Servings: 8

Ingredients:
- 2 tablespoons butter
- 4 lbs. double beef brisket, trimmed
- 2 onions, thinly sliced
- 5 garlic cloves, minced
- 4 celery stalks, diced
- 1 tablespoon ground cumin
- 2 teaspoons dried oregano
- 1 cinnamon stick
- 1 teaspoon cracked black peppercorns
- ½ teaspoon of sea salt
- 1 can tomatoes with juice
- 1 cup chicken stock
- 2 cups boiling water
- 3 dried guajillo chilies
- 1 jalapeño pepper, diced
- 1 cup cilantro
- 1 green bell pepper, diced

Directions:

1. Heat oil in a skillet. Add brisket and cook for 6 minutes or until brown on all sides. Transfer into the slow cooker.
2. Add remaining butter. Cook onions, garlic, celery, cumin, oregano, cinnamon stick, peppercorns, and sea salt. Stir well. Add tomatoes with juice, stock, and water. Bring to a boil.
3. Transfer all ingredients into the slow cooker. Cover the lid and cook on low for 8 hours.
4. Soak chilies. Cook for another 30 minutes. Discard stems and soaking liquid.
5. Transfer mixture into a blender. Add jalapeño and cilantro. Puree and add into the slow cooker. Add bell pepper.
6. Reposition the lid and cook on high for 20 minutes. Serve.

146. STEWED OXTAILS

Prep Time: 15 mins
Total Time: 2 hrs. 15 mins
Total Time: 2 hours 30 mins
Servings: 8

Ingredients:
- 2 tablespoons clarified butter
- 4 lbs. oxtails, cut into 2-inch pieces
- 2 onions, finely chopped
- 3 garlic cloves, minced
- 2 celery stalks, diced
- 2 carrots, diced
- 1 teaspoon dried thyme leaves
- ½ teaspoon of sea salt
- ½ Cracked black peppercorns
- 1 bay leaf
- 1 ½ cups dry red wine
- 1 can tomatoes with juice
- 12 oz. mushrooms, quartered
- 1.2 cup parsley leaves, finely chopped

Directions:
1. Heat 1 tablespoon of butter in a skillet. Cook oxtails, in batches, and cook for 4 minutes or until lightly browned all over. Transfer into the slow cooker.
2. Add remaining butter. Cook onions, garlic, celery, carrots, thyme, sea, salt, peppercorns, and bay leaf. Stir well.

3. Pour wine and bring to a boil. Scrape brown bits from the bottom of the pan. Add tomatoes with juice.
4. Transfer all ingredients into the slow cooker. Add mushrooms. Cover the lid and cook on low for 8 hours. Discard bay leaves. Garnish with parsley.

147. POT ROAST

Prep Time: 15 mins
Total Time: 2 hrs. 15 mins
Total Time: 2 hours 30 mins
Servings: 8

Ingredients:
- 2 tablespoons clarified butter
- 2 oz. pancetta, diced
- 2 onions, finely chopped
- 4 garlic cloves, minced
- 2 celery stalks, diced
- 2 carrots, diced
- 1 teaspoon dried rosemary leaves
- 2 bay leaves
- 1 cinnamon stick
- ½ teaspoon of sea salt
- ½ teaspoon cracked black peppercorns
- 2 tablespoons tomato paste
- 3 cups red wine
- Pinch of sea salt
- Pinch of ground black pepper

Directions:
1. Heat 1 tablespoon clarified butter in a skillet. Cook pancetta for 3 minutes on each side until browned. Transfer into the slow cooker.
2. Add beef and cook for 8 minutes or until brown on all sides. Transfer into the slow cooker.
3. In the same skillet, add remaining clarified butter. Sauté onion, garlic, celery, carrots, rosemary, bay leaves, cinnamon stick, sea salt, and peppercorns. Stir in tomato paste. Pour wine. Stir well. Bring to a boil.
4. Transfer into the slow cooker. Cover the lid and cook on low for 8 hours.
5. Transfer meat to a platter. Keep warm. Discard bay leaves. Puree sauce using an immersion blender. Adjust taste if needed. Slice meat and serve.

148. Oxtails with Celery

Prep Time: 30 mins
Cook Time: 3 hrs.
Total Time: 3 hrs. 30 mins
Servings: 6

Ingredients:
- 2 tablespoons olive oil, divided
- 4 oz. pancetta, diced
- 4 lbs. oxtails cut into 2-inch pieces
- 1 onion , diced
- 2 garlic cloves, minced
- 2 celery stalks, diced
- 1 teaspoon of sea salt
- 1 teaspoon black peppercorns
- 1 cup dry white wine
- 1 cup tomato paste
- 2 cups chicken stock
- 6 cups celery, sliced
- ½ cup parsley cloves, finely chopped

Directions:
1. Heat olive oil in a skillet Add pancetta and cook for 4 minutes until browned on all sides. Transfer into the slow cooker.
2. Add oxtails, and cook in batches, for 5 minutes or until brown on all sides. Transfer into the slow cooker.
3. Heat the remaining oil. Sauté onion, garlic, celery, sea salt, and peppercorns for 4 minutes. Pour wine. Scrape up brown bits. Stir in tomato paste and chicken stock.
4. Transfer into the slow cooker. Cover the lid and cook on low for 8 hours.
5. When oxtails are almost cooked, bring a pot with salted water to a boil. Add celery and oxtails. Transfer into the slow cooker again. Cover and cook on high for 10 minutes. Garnish with parsley. Serve.

149. Italian- Style Goulash

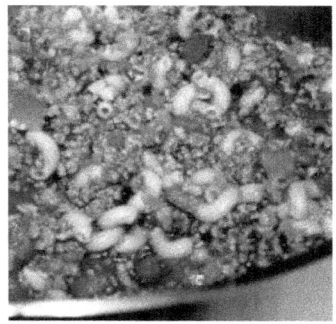

Prep Time: 20 mins
Cook Time: 1 hrs.
Total Time: 1 hrs. 20 mins
Servings: 4

Ingredients:
- 2 tablespoons olive oil
- 2 lbs. stewing beef, trimmed
- 2 onions, diced
- 2 garlic cloves, minced
- 2 celery stalks, diced
- 1 carrot, diced
- 2 teaspoons dried oregano
- 1 teaspoon dried rosemary
- ½ teaspoon of sea salt
- 1.2 teaspoon cracked black peppercorns
- ¼ cup tomato paste
- 1 cup dry red wine
- 2 potatoes, diced
- 2 cups beef stock
- 1 teaspoon hot paprika
- 1 tablespoon sweet paprika
- 2 tablespoons water

Directions:
1. Heat oil in a skillet. Cook beef, in batches, for 5 minutes or until lightly browned. Transfer into the slow cooker.
2. Heat the remaining oil. Sauté onion, garlic, celery, carrot, oregano, rosemary, sea salt, and peppercorns for 7 minutes. Stir in tomato paste. Pour wine. Bring to a boil. Scrape up brown bits from the bottom of the pan. Transfer into the slow cooker.
3. Add potatoes and pour stock. Cover the lid and cook on low for 8 hours.

4. Meanwhile, in a bowl, dissolve hot and sweet paprika in water. Stir well. Add to the slow cooker. Reposition the lid. Cover and cook on high for 15 minutes. Serve.

150. Coco Ginger Linguine

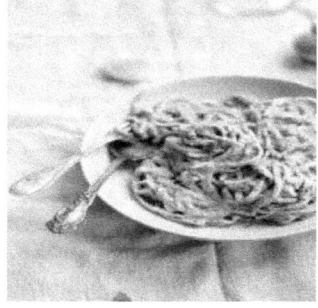

Prep Time: 15 mins
Cook Time: 15 mins
Total Time: 30 mins
Servings: 6

Ingredients:
- 8 oz. dry linguine
- 1 cup spinach leaves, rinsed and drained
- ½ cup Swiss chard, rinsed and dried
- ½ tbsp. olive oil
- 2 small garlic cloves, minced
- 1 ½ tbsps. fresh ginger, grated
- 8 oz. coconut milk
- ¼ tsp. stevia
- 1 ½ tsps. lemon juice, freshly squeezed
- Red pepper flakes
- Sea salt

- ❖ Ground black pepper

Directions:
1. Cook the pasta based on the package instructions. Rinse over cold water, drain thoroughly, and set aside.
2. Meanwhile, place garlic, ginger, stevia, coconut milk in the slow cooker. Mix well. Season with red pepper flakes, salt, and pepper. Add spinach and Swiss chard. Cover the lid. Cook on low for 4 hours.
3. Let cool, and then pour into a blender or food processor. Blend until creamy.
4. Transfer the pasta into a serving bowl, and then add the sauce. Toss well to coat, and then serve right away.

151. VEGAN MACARONI AND CHEESE

Prep Time: 15 mins
Cook Time: 25 mins
Total Time: 40 mins
Servings: 4

Ingredients:
- ❖ 6 oz. whole wheat rotini
- ❖ 2 ½ tbsps nutritional yeast
- ❖ 2 ½ tbsps non-dairy butter
- ❖ ½ panko breadcrumbs
- ❖ 1 cup broccoli, chopped, steamed
- ❖ ½ cup sweet potato, diced
- ❖ ½ carrot, diced
- ❖ ½ cup water
- ❖ ½ tbsp. miso paste
- ❖ ½ tbsp. lemon juice, freshly squeezed
- ❖ ½ tbsp. tahini
- ❖ ½ tsp. Dijon mustard
- ❖ 2 tbsps. cashews, chopped
- ❖ ½ tsp. sea salt

Directions:
1. Cook the pasta based on the package instructions. Rinse over cold water, drain thoroughly, and set aside.

2. In a slow cooker, combine carrot and sweet potato. Add the remaining ingredients, except for breadcrumbs and pasta. Cover the lid. Cook on low for 4 hours.
3. Allow to cool and then transfer in a food processor. Blend until smooth.
4. Transfer in a casserole dish. Top with the panko breadcrumbs. Bake for 15 minutes, or until the top is golden brown. Best served warm.

152. GLAZED SALMON

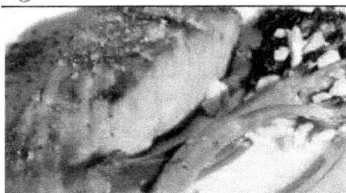

Prep Time: 15 mins
Cook Time: 5 mins
Total Time: 1 hr. 20 mins
Servings: 6

Ingredients:
- ¼ cup soy sauce, reduced-sodium
- 1 tbsp. lime juice
- 2 tbsps. syrup, ample
- 2 tbsps. scallions, chopped
- 4 fillets, salmon
- 1 tbsp. ginger, freshly grated

Directions:
1. Mix soy sauce, maple syrup, and lime juice in a mixing bowl. Add scallions and ginger, stirring well to combine. Stir in the salmon fillets and coat well with the mixture.
2. Transfer in the slow cooker. Cover the lid and cook on low for 6 hours. Best served warm.

153. STROGANOFF

Prep Time: 15 mins
Cook Time: 15 mins
Total Tim: 30 mins
Servings: 8

Ingredients:
- 8 oz. mushrooms, cremini, sliced
- ½ cup shallots, chopped
- 1 tablespoon cornstarch, mixed w/ ¼ cup water
- ¾ pound steak, top round, w/ fat trimmed
- 1 ¼ cups beef broth, low-sodium, fat-free
- 1 tablespoon mustard, Dijon
- 4 servings noodles, wide, cooked
- ½ cup yoghurt, plain, low-fat

Directions:
1. Slice beef into extremely thin slices, cut into bite-sized pieces. Transfer in the slow cooker.
2. Add in mushrooms, shallots, broth, mustard, cornstarch, and yoghurt. Stir well. Cover the lid and cook on low for 2 hours.
3. Serve over hot noodles.

154. BARLEY AND SQUASH CROCKPOT

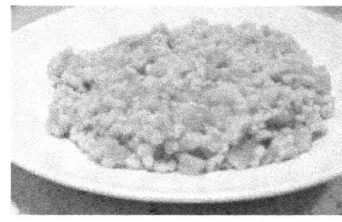

Prep Time: 15 mins
Cook Time: 3 hrs. 30 mins
Total Time: 3 hours 45 mins
Servings: 6

Ingredients:
- 1 tbsp. olive oil
- 1tbsp. non-dairy butter
- ½ cup pearl barley
- 1 ¾ cups butternut squash, cubed
- 1 garlic clove, minced
- ½ red onion, minced
- 1 tbsp. whole wheat flour
- 1 cup non-dairy milk

- ❖ 1 tsp. dried rosemary
- ❖ ½ cup non-dairy cheddar cheese, shredded
- ❖ 1/3 cup Parmesan cheese, shredded
- ❖ Nutmeg
- ❖ ¼ tsp. sea salt
- ❖ Ground black pepper

Directions:
1. Combine water and barley in the slow cooker. Add garlic, onion, squash, butter, flour, milk, rosemary, and a dash of nutmeg in the slow cooker. Season to taste with salt and pepper.
2. Cover the lid and cook on low for 2 hours.
3. Mix the squash, barley and sauce in a baking dish, then top with Parmesan cheese. Seal with aluminum foil and bake for 15 minutes.
4. Uncover and set the oven to broil. Broil for 3 minutes, or until the casserole is golden brown. Let cool for 10 minutes, and then serve.

155. SEITAN IN TOMATO AND SOY YOGURT

Prep Time: 5 mins
Cook Time: 20 mins
Total Time: 25 mins
Servings: 6

Ingredients:
- ❖ ½ lb. seitan
- ❖ 1 onion, diced
- ❖ 2 garlic cloves
- ❖ 2 ½ tbsps soy yoghurt
- ❖ 2 ½ tbsps tomato sauce
- ❖ ½ tsp. cumin
- ❖ ¼ tsp. cayenne pepper
- ❖ 1 fresh clove
- ❖ ½ tsp. sea salt

Directions:
1. Slice seitan into bite-sized cubes and set aside.
2. If using wooden skewers, soak them in cold water.
3. Combine yoghurt, tomato sauce, onion, garlic, cumin, cayenne, and clove in the slow cooker. Cover the lid and cook on low for 2 hours.
4. Allow to cool and then pour in a food processor. Blend until smooth.

5. Transfer mixture into a bowl, and then place the seitan in it. Turn to coat. Best served warm.

156. CRANBERRY-APPLE PORK

Prep Time: 15 mins
Cook Time: 8 hrs.
Total Time: 8 hrs. 15 mins
Servings: 6

Ingredients:
- 2 apples, Granny Smith, peeled, cored, sliced thickly
- 1 tablespoon sugar, brown
- 1 cup cranberries, fresh
- 2 pork tenderloins, one-pounder, w/ sliver skin and fat trimmed
- ½ cup cider
- 2 tablespoons cider vinegar
- 1 teaspoon cinnamon

Directions:
1. Place tenderloins inside the slow cooker. Arrange apple slices around the pork. Scatter cranberries.
2. Pour in cider vinegar and apple cider, and then dust the surface of the pork with cinnamon and sugar.
3. Cover the lid and cook on low for 8 hours. Let stand for ten minutes. Serve.

157. HERBED TENDERLOIN

Prep Time: 5 mins.
Cook Time: 40 mins.
Total Time: 45 mins
Servings: 12

Ingredients:
- ¾ cup pork tenderloin
- ¼ cup mixed herbs (thyme, parsley, rosemary, sage), fresh, chopped finely
- ½ teaspoon black pepper, freshly ground

Directions:

1. Coat pork with the herbs. Tuck in thin ends to make sure the pork evenly cooks.
2. Place pork in the slow cooker. Cover the lid and cook on low for 8 hours or on high for 4 hours.
3. Let stand for ten minutes. Serve.

158. CORN AND MUSHROOM

Prep Time: 5 mins
Cook Time: 15 mins
Total Time: 20 mins
Servings: 4

Ingredients:
- 2 Tbsps. vegetable stock, unsalted
- 1 can, 15 oz. button mushrooms, pieces and stems, rinsed, drained
- 1 Tbsp. coconut oil, organic
- 2 cans, 15 oz. each whole corn kernels, rinsed, drained
- 1 shallot, peeled, minced
- salt
- white pepper, to taste

Directions:
1. Pour ingredients into the slow cooker. Pour stock until liquid reaches 4-cup line of the pot. Stir.
2. Cover the lid and cook on low for 4 hours.
3. Divide into equal portions. Serve

159. THAI TOFU BOWLS

Prep Time: 20mins
Cook Time10mins
Total Time 30 mins
Servings: 4

Ingredients:
- ½ tsp olive oil
- 24 oz. extra firm tofu, cubed

- ❖ 1 ½ cups vegetable broth
- ❖ 1 cup cauliflower, chopped
- ❖ 3 tbsps. scallions, chopped
- ❖ 1 garlic clove, crushed
- ❖ ¼ cup onion, chopped
- ❖ 1 tsp. ginger grated
- ❖ 1 celery stalk, sliced
- ❖ ½ tbsp. lemon juice, freshly squeezed
- ❖ ½ tsp. five-spice
- ❖ 1/ tsp hot pepper sauce
- ❖ ¼ tsp sea salt
- ❖ 3 tbsps. fresh cilantro, chopped

Directions:
1. Place tofu cubes in the slow cooker. Add onion, garlic, celery, lemon juice, salt, ginger, and five-spice. Mix well.
2. Stir hot pepper sauce in the broth until thoroughly combined, and then pour into the slow cooker. Shred cauliflower in the food processor until grainy. Put inside the slow cooker.
3. Cover the lid and cook on low for 4 hours.
4. Divide mixture among bowls. Garnish with cilantro. Serve.

160. BEEF WITH MUSHROOMS AND SWEET POTATO

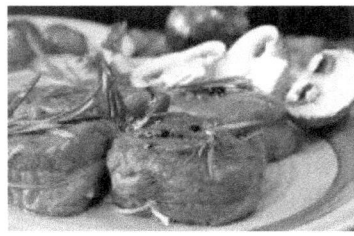

Prep time: 20 mins
Cook time: 1 hour 10 mins
Total time: 1 hour 30 mins
Servings: 6

Ingredients:
- ❖ 2/3 lb. stewing beef, lean
- ❖ 8 oz. button mushrooms, halved
- ❖ 1 cup red wine
- ❖ 1 onion, roughly chopped

- ❖ 2 bay leaves
- ❖ 2 celery stalks, sliced
- ❖ 1 tsp. dried thyme
- ❖ 2 cups sweet potato, chopped
- ❖ 2 tbsps. tomato paste
- ❖ 1 garlic clove, crushed
- ❖ 8 oz. tomato sauce, w/out added salt
- ❖ 2 carrots, sliced
- ❖ 15 oz. black beans, reduced-sodium, drained, rinsed
- ❖ 1 tsp. dried oregano

Directions:
1. Fill the slow cooker with vegetables before adding in the beef. Pour red wine, bay leaves, black beans, tomato sauce, tomato paste, and herbs.
2. Cover the lid. Allow the mixture to cook for eight hours on low. Serve.

CONCLUSION

There is a large body of evidence which supports the role of inflammation in the pathophysiology of mental health disorders, including depression. Dietary patterns have been shown to modulate the inflammatory state, thus highlighting their potential as a therapeutic tool in disorders with an inflammatory basis.

It is a well-known fact that different foods are metabolized differently, some promoting inflammation and others reducing it. The purpose of the anti-inflammatory diet is to promote optimal health and healing by choosing foods that reduce inflammation. If one can successfully control excessive inflammation through natural means (like through diet), it reduces one's dependence on anti-inflammatory medications that have unwanted and unhealthy side effects and don't solve the underlying problem. While anti-inflammatory medications (such as NSAIDs) are a quick fix to ease symptoms, they ultimately weaken the immune system by damaging the gastrointestinal tract which plays an important role in immune system function.

www.ingramcontent.com/pod-product-compliance
Lightning Source LLC
Chambersburg PA
CBHW070633220526
45466CB00001B/166